# THE BOOK OF MAID

# THE BOOK OF MAID

## Understanding Medical Assistance in Dying in Canada

GEORGE S. TAKACH

sh.
SUTHERLAND HOUSE

TORONTO, 2026

Sutherland House
416 Moore Ave., Suite 304
Toronto, ON M4G 1C9



First edition, August 2026

If you are interested in inviting one of our authors to a live event or media appearance, please contact sranasinghe@sutherlandhousebooks.com and visit our website at sutherlandhousebooks.com for more information about our authors and their schedules.

Manufactured in Canada
Cover designed by Leah Ciani and Jordan Lunn
Book composed by Karl Hunt

Library and Archives Canada Cataloguing in Publication
Title: The book of MAID : understanding medically assisted dying in Canada / George Takach.
Names: Takach, George S. (George Steven), author
Description: First edition.
Identifiers: Canadiana (print) 20260190772 | Canadiana (ebook) 20260190799 | ISBN 9781997701798 (softcover) | ISBN 9781997701804 (EPUB)
Subjects: LCSH: Assisted suicide—Canada. | CSH: Medical assistance in dying—Canada.
Classification: LCC R726 .T35 2026 | DDC 179.7—dc23

ISBN 978-1-997701-79-8
eBook 978-1-997701-80-4

For Barb—I learn so much
from you every day.

Also by George S. Takach

*Contracting for Computers*

*The Software Business*

*Computer Law*

*Cold War 2.0: Artificial Intelligence in the New Battle Between China, Russia and America*

*Inspired by Taiwan*

# CONTENTS

# INTRODUCTION

You've just received difficult medical news. Perhaps your cancer has returned, and this time it's incurable. Or your chronic medical condition has progressed, and the next phase will involve a serious decline in your independence. In either case, or a similar circumstance, you may be wondering how medical assistance in dying (MAID) might factor in, and what it might mean in practical terms. Alternatively, you might have a family member or close friend who has just shared such news with you, and who, at the end of the conversation, began asking questions about MAID.

Faced with one of these situations, you've decided to learn more about MAID in Canada. When do people use it? How does it work? What do you tell your family and friends, especially if you're unsure how they'll react? If so, this book is for you. It's a practical guide to MAID, designed to quickly equip you with the knowledge to speak effectively with healthcare professionals and loved ones. You'll also find a curated guide to MAID resources. Remember, you don't have to consider MAID alone—experienced people are ready to help.

## The Essential Promise of MAID

In Canada, if you have a serious and incurable medical condition that has caused advanced, irreversible decline, resulting in intolerable suffering, and you meet certain other criteria and safeguards, then, entirely at your discretion, you can ask a doctor or nurse practitioner to end your life with dignity and compassion through medical assistance in dying.

This is the core promise of MAID in Canada: if a medical condition is causing you great suffering, you are entitled to request MAID, provided you meet specific criteria. Currently, roughly 15,000 Canadians each year choose MAID. This book draws upon their experiences to present a practical guide.

## Why Do People Choose MAID?

The 76,475 Canadians who chose MAID up to the end of 2024 (the latest statistics available before this book went to press) expressed a wide range of reasons. They all had serious and incurable medical conditions, were in an advanced state of decline, and experienced intolerable suffering. Their reasons may well resonate with you.

Some specifically cited a diminished quality of life compared to their previous experiences. Others said they were no longer able to enjoy life. Others highlighted a loss of dignity or independence. Some emphasized a desire to avoid being a burden on others. Some couldn't bear the pain, despite trying various pain relief medications and palliative care. Still others, suffering from dementia or Alzheimer's, mourned the loss of memory and cognitive ability, fearing the inevitable worsening had they not chosen MAID. Other MAID recipients offer further reasons.

If you choose MAID, it may be for similar reasons, or for entirely different ones. While all MAID recipients share three conditions—a serious incurable medical condition, an advanced state of decline, and intolerable suffering—every MAID experience is intensely personal. Should you elect to have MAID, your reasons will reflect your unique circumstances, but may also echo the experiences of the tens of thousands of Canadians who have chosen MAID before you. This book shares some of their experiences, hoping to help you contemplate your own circumstances.

## MAID as a Consolation

You may be reading this not because you have an incurable medical condition, but because someone close to you does. When a family member or close friend chooses MAID, you will likely feel deep, profound sadness and grieve their death. However, MAID may also offer a silver lining in this difficult situation.

Your loved one chose MAID because they were suffering intolerably. Remember what drove them to this decision: the end-stage cancer causing constant pain, or the dementia steadily eroding their memory and cognitive ability, causing existential suffering at the thought of no longer recognizing loved ones, including you. Ultimately, it is the debilitating, serious, and incurable medical condition that warrants your sadness. Life can be cruel in that the dying process, or a certain point in a person's chronic disease, disability, or medical condition, can cause so much suffering.

For some facing such profound suffering, MAID offers significant relief. It allows your family member or friend to avoid the worst suffering that would otherwise occur without the option of MAID. This is why MAID providers (doctors or nurse practitioners) offer this service: they help patients face and overcome the extreme suffering caused by a serious and incurable medical condition. MAID patients invariably thank their providers just before the procedure, which consoles the provider and instills pride in their work. As you face losing a loved one to a cruel and painful disease, this compassionate reality of MAID may also be consoling to you.

## Important Disclaimer

This book is a general introduction to MAID. Decisions around MAID can be complicated, involving personal factors, detailed medical considerations, and legal aspects. This book provides only a general overview of the issues involved. No book (or internet source or AI program) can accurately answer all your questions about MAID. If you are considering MAID in Canada, you need to speak with a MAID provider. Information on how to contact a MAID provider is available at the end of Chapter 3.

## The Flow of This Book

Your first question about MAID might well be: "When can I even consider it?" Chapter 1, therefore, discusses when MAID might make sense. To illustrate how people often think about MAID, Chapter 1 includes several "MAID journeys." High-profile Canadian businessperson Tim Hockey recounts the MAID stories of his father and wife, both involving end-of-life cancer. Tim's story is particularly relevant because two-thirds of Canadians who access MAID do so to avoid further suffering from end-of-life cancer. Another MAID story in Chapter 1 is about renowned Canadian children's book author Robert Munsch. Media reports discuss his decision to have MAID due to dementia and Parkinson's; he told the *New York Times* that he does not want to reach the point where he no longer recognizes his loved ones or can communicate. This case is also relevant, as about 770,000 Canadians have dementia of some kind (about 65 percent due to Alzheimer's), and approximately 62,500 new dementia patients are diagnosed each year in Canada.

MAID involves an incredibly personal decision, but it generally also involves family and friends. Chapter 2, therefore, discusses potentially sensitive issues involving your loved ones. If you decide to have MAID, how might you approach your closest family members? Or perhaps you are the spouse, son, daughter (or other family member or close friend) of someone who has elected to have MAID; how will you respond to their news? It's worth thinking about these questions in advance. Chapter 2 offers suggestions you may find helpful.

The nuances of MAID can be confusing. Chapter 3, therefore, provides the essentials: When can you have MAID? How do you qualify? What medical conditions does MAID apply to? What safeguards must you satisfy? Chapter 3 also explains the different steps of the MAID process in Canada. While this chapter won't answer all your questions, it will help you understand how MAID works in Canada.

In essence, Chapters 1–3 give you the practical "basics" about MAID in Canada. You will likely find your key immediate questions discussed in these chapters, especially if you are responding to difficult medical news of your own or from a loved one. You may, however, have additional questions. Chapter 4 discusses how Canada arrived at its MAID system. Chapter 5 covers some current unresolved issues around MAID that legislators and courts in Canada continue to consider. While you are likely most curious about successful MAID requests, you might also find it useful to know why so many MAID requests are refused or unfulfilled—that is the subject of Chapter 6. Finally, if you're looking to explore additional material about MAID (beyond the information at the end of Chapter 3 related to finding a MAID provider and a MAID support group), Chapter 7 has a curated list of resources.

## It's Entirely Your Choice

One last (but important) point: whether you decide to have MAID or not is solely *your choice*. Moreover, there is no right or wrong answer—there is merely your personal preference. Some people diagnosed with end-of-life cancer (where a natural death is reasonably foreseeable) want to fight to their last breath, enduring excruciating suffering, including (for example) months of difficult chemotherapy to gain an extra twelve months of life. Others, particularly if elderly, don't think this path makes sense and choose MAID (often after a period of palliative care). Some people with Multiple Sclerosis decide that when their bowel and bladder no longer function properly, they opt for MAID to stop their suffering. Others in the same stage of MS accept the accommodations their medical condition requires, including eventually using a colostomy bag. Essentially, MAID will not be everyone's choice, but it is comforting to know that in Canada it's an option, a potential choice, but always one that is up to you.

# CHAPTER 1

# WHEN TO CONSIDER MAID

Before delving into the practical aspects of MAID and the related personal considerations, it's important to discuss the circumstances under which MAID might be considered. This chapter outlines four scenarios where MAID may seem like a reasonable option:

1. You are experiencing a significant decline due to a terminal illness and are suffering greatly.
2. You have experienced a debilitating stroke or accident, resulting in irreversible decline and significant suffering.
3. You have a neurodegenerative disease, leading to irreversible decline and significant suffering.
4. You have dementia, resulting in irreversible decline and significant suffering.

You may be reading this book because you are currently facing one of these situations, or someone you love is. Alternatively, you may be considering MAID as a logical extension of end-of-life planning, even if you don't have an immediate medical crisis. Ideally, you have already prepared a will and an Advance Directive for other medical decisions. Regardless, this chapter will provide insight into the kinds of life events that can prompt serious consideration of MAID.

## A Reminder about Human Suffering

Before examining the four scenarios mentioned earlier, it's worth reflecting on the nature of the human body. It's a marvel of science, evolution, and increasingly, modern medicine. While we've made significant progress in understanding the biology, chemistry, and medicine that sustain life, the human body remains incredibly complex, fragile, and ultimately finite.

Since the dawn of Homo sapiens, the arc of human life has generally followed a similar pattern: birth in a state of helplessness, followed by physical, mental, intellectual, and emotional growth nurtured by others. Physical strength peaks in the twenties, and then, around the early thirties, the body's 7,500 individual parts begin to decline, slowly at first. If you're fortunate enough to reach your sixtieth birthday, this decline often accelerates. By your seventies and eighties, serious malfunctions of various body parts, including brain degeneration, can become overwhelming, unless illness or disease has already ended your life.

One of the cruel ironies of aging is that our organs decline at different rates. When the brain develops dementia, it doesn't signal the heart and lungs to shut down. Even with severe cognitive decay, the heart continues to beat, and the lungs continue to breathe, often for years. They remain oblivious to the tragedy unfolding in the brain.

Conversely, nerve degeneration, as in ALS or MS, can cause muscle failure and physical collapse, while the brain remains sharp. The mind is then forced to witness the body's agonizing decline, a torment that could be avoided if all organs failed simultaneously. Instead, each organ's semi-autonomous function and unique decline schedule compounds suffering.

Adding to this hardship is the burden placed on loved ones—spouses, children, siblings, parents, and friends—who must witness the decline. These experiences leave them with painful, indelible memories. In their minds, images of suffering often overshadow happier recollections.

With the average Canadian now living to nearly eighty-two, most deaths result from the failure of one or more bodily systems. The surprise isn't that the body eventually wears out, but that it functions so well for so long. Consider the heart, which beats roughly 100,000 times a day, totalling an astounding 3.15 billion times over a lifetime. Given this incredible workload, it's no wonder heart problems are a leading cause of death.

We are all mortal, and our lives will inevitably end, often with some degree of suffering. A key personal consideration is how that end will unfold, including the extent of suffering during the dying process. Alternatively, you may already be experiencing significant decline and suffering due to a chronic condition. The following sections discuss four potential end-of-life scenarios or the progression of serious chronic conditions. Consider whether MAID could play a role in mitigating suffering in these circumstances, either by avoiding it altogether or significantly reducing it.

## Scenario 1: Avoiding Further Suffering from the Dying Process

The only certainty in life is death, preceded by a period of decline, or the "dying process." Like the 109 billion people who have lived and died on Earth over the past 300,000 years, you too will eventually cease to breathe, your heart will stop, and your brain will no longer function. Death, preceded by a dying process, is inevitable.

In Canada today, most people die from end-stage cancer, fatal heart or lung disease, catastrophic organ failure, or another incurable illness or "end-of-life" condition where natural death is reasonably foreseeable. As a complex system of interconnected parts, your body will gradually decline, and in the final months, you may find yourself more "dying" than "living." This period constitutes the dying process.

The dying process can last months or weeks, depending on the underlying medical condition and the degree of organ decline. During this time, you will likely experience considerable discomfort and pain as bodily functions begin to shut down. This can lead to complications, including bowel and bladder issues, breathing or heart problems, severe fatigue, and exhaustion.

For example, the dying process in the final weeks of end-stage cancer (where natural death is reasonably foreseeable) often includes some or all of the following:

- Withdrawal: loss of interest in previously enjoyed activities, reduced social engagement, irritability, and restlessness.
- Drowsiness: increased sleep, difficulty waking, falling asleep during conversations, and tiring easily during visits.

The following conditions may arise:

- Difficulty swallowing: problems swallowing can lead to choking or increase the risk of lung infection if forced to eat.
- Laboured breathing: breathing may become irregular (mucus can pool in the throat, causing a gurgling sound that may distress visitors).

- Bowel and bladder problems: incontinence may occur due to loss of bowel and bladder control from weakened pelvic muscles; this may require the use of a catheter for urine and diapers for bowel movements.
- Skin conditions: the skin may become thin and translucent, sometimes with red blotches.
- Delirium: restlessness and confusion may manifest as disorientation (not knowing the day or location), hallucinations, frustration, fear, agitation, or even physical aggression; speech may become garbled; these symptoms, collectively known as delirium, resemble advanced dementia but develop rapidly; erratic, involuntary movements of the arms and legs may also occur, which can be upsetting to family and friends.

Consider the final stage of the dying process experienced by Tanner Martin, age thirty, as described in the *Washington Post* article “Life Was Awesome”:

> Alongside medications to ease his nausea and anxiety, doctors turned to their most powerful drugs to quiet his body’s distress—fentanyl, ketamine, haldol, morphine, dilaudid—in various combinations. Nothing helped. Tanner’s pain grew sharper each day, and he was throwing up constantly. Every few hours the cycle repeated: strip the sheets, strip his clothes, clean him up, wait for it to happen again.

Between June 15, 2025, and June 24, 2025, his parents were so shaken that they texted their extended family asking for prayers for Tanner’s swift and peaceful passing. Tanner died on June 25, 2025.

For Canadians contemplating their own end-of-life experience, a fundamental question arises: do I want to risk experiencing a situation like Tanner’s? Do I want to reach a point where my religious family is praying for my swift and painless death? Beyond the immediate physical discomfort, there is the suffering caused by anticipating worsening pain and discomfort, knowing that, unlike other medical interventions, there is no cure, only death after an awful, painful, and suffering-filled dying process. In other words, concerns may not be about death itself, but rather the dying process.

In Canada, individuals facing the dying process have several options, which can be pursued individually or in combination. First, one can choose to allow the natural course of dying to unfold without intervention, as exemplified by Tanner's fate in the aforementioned excerpt. Some religious perspectives view suffering as ennobling, and those who hold this belief may opt not to alleviate the pain and suffering inherent in the dying process. Instead, they allow events to unfold naturally, foregoing steps, such as MAID, to hasten death. In essence, they endure the suffering inherent in the dying process. Actively refusing MAID is unnecessary, as a natural death is the default under Canadian law; inaction results in a "natural death." To access MAID, an individual must actively choose it and take the necessary steps. Absent the choice of MAID or palliative care, the dying process will be a traditional, natural one, culminating in a natural death.

The second option is palliative care, overseen by a palliative care physician. In this approach, the medical focus shifts from curing or treating the underlying condition to maximizing comfort by addressing symptoms, particularly pain management through medication. Palliative care can be administered at home, in a hospital, or increasingly in a hospice setting. Hospices provide specialized care during the final weeks of life, with professionals dedicated to ensuring comfort.

Many Canadians find palliative care sufficient to meet their end-of-life needs, and thankfully, its coverage within Canada's healthcare system has expanded in recent decades. However, some Canadians find that palliative care does not address all their end-of-life concerns. Notably, approximately 75 percent of Canadians who choose MAID each year are already receiving palliative care. Specifically, palliative care may not alleviate fears of loss of dignity or shield family members from the distressing aspects of palliative sedation, which can involve involuntary convulsions and groans as bodily functions gradually cease. Many believe that the final stages of palliative care can lead to an undignified death, and often, by the time this becomes apparent to the patient, it may be too late to pursue MAID.

A third option, available in Canada for about a decade, is MAID, which allows you to avoid suffering through the final stages of a natural death. You might choose MAID to spare your family the difficult physical and emotional scenes that can accompany the dying process, avoiding a situation like the Tanner situation described earlier.

MAID and palliative care are often viewed as complementary choices. Quebec's MAID law, for example, addresses both as complementary services within "end-of-life care." You may begin your end-of-life journey with palliative care and find it sufficient for the entire process. However, if palliative care, or palliative care alone, cannot meet your end-of-life goals, you may choose MAID.

If your serious and incurable medical condition causes intolerable suffering, and you meet the criteria and safeguards discussed in Chapter 3, a MAID provider can administer medication to allow you to die peacefully, painlessly, and with compassion and dignity. You can choose to be surrounded by family and friends at a time of your choosing. MAID effectively shortens the dying process, avoiding much of the pain and suffering that might otherwise consume your final weeks or months. It can also alleviate concerns about being a burden on your family, a significant consideration for many MAID requesters (as noted in Chapter 3, 49 percent of requesters in 2024 feared being a burden).

While MAID cannot eliminate suffering altogether—eligibility requires already experiencing intolerable suffering—it can significantly reduce its duration.

Furthermore, MAID allows you to choose the date and time of its provision. This provides ample time to say farewell to loved ones, perhaps hold a celebration of life with a wider circle of friends, and generally ensure your affairs are in order. With MAID, you can also better ensure that appropriate words are exchanged, and hugs given, to those who matter most. You also have the opportunity to make amends with those with whom you have fallen out, all while you still have sufficient energy and endurance to say goodbye properly.

To illustrate how MAID can be used to manage the dying process, consider the experiences of David Hockey, as recounted by his son, Tim Hockey, a well-known Canadian businessperson. Tim spent thirty-two years at TD Bank, rising to the number three position and running its retail banking division, Canada's largest branch network. He later served as CEO of TD Ameritrade, the successful online brokerage based in New York.

David, who bore an uncanny resemblance to John Cleese of Monty Python fame, was a serious man, despite the comedian's humour. Over his eighty-seven years, David was a scientist, teacher, philosopher, and more. A humanist and a pragmatic Brit, he emigrated to Canada in the 1950s to "provide a better future for his family," according to his obituary.

"When my dad was diagnosed with metastasizing prostate cancer," Tim recounts, "he chose not to pursue chemo or other invasive treatments that would only extend his life a little. Instead, he focused on living a busy life for as long as he could."

David's approach to his own death was influenced by his experiences caring for his wife and sister at home as they succumbed to cancer in the pre-MAID era. "My dad didn't want to end his life the way my mom and aunt had, now that he could choose a different route with MAID," Tim explains.

A fall that resulted in a broken collarbone proved to be the turning point for David. While recuperating in an Ottawa hospital, he called his son in Toronto to share his decision. "We spoke regularly by phone, about an hour a day, and all of a sudden my dad tells me he's going to have MAID. I was a little surprised, but on reflection it made total sense for him. He was a very rational man. Once he concluded that his suffering didn't buy him enough pleasure in life, MAID was a logical route for his final cancer journey. He also took great pride in being a provider for his family, and he refused to be a burden on his family, including his partner Anne, who had been in his life since my mother passed away. My dad viewed MAID as the most natural thing to do in his predicament."

The day before David's MAID procedure, his immediate family gathered in Ottawa to say their goodbyes. Though tears were shed, the atmosphere was largely one of fond remembrance. David's children (including Tim and his two older sisters), grandchildren, and great-grandchildren were all present. During the gathering, one of the grandchildren drove to the cabin on Rideau Lake, north of Ottawa, that David had purchased in the 1960s. The family had spent countless hours there throughout the years. Although the cottage was no longer in the family, the grandchild persuaded the current owner to allow a brief FaceTime call to David from inside. It was a surprise treat that David and the others thoroughly enjoyed, sparking a flood of memories. One of the benefits of MAID, when well-managed, is that it allows the patient to create the time and space for family to gather, say goodbye, experience an important milestone together, and begin grieving collectively.

The next day, for the MAID procedure, only David, his three children, Anne (the MAID nurse who inserted the IV line), and Dr. Casey (who would administer the medication) were present. After the IV was in place, David, channelling his inner John Cleese, joked, "I guess I'll have to go ahead with this now, or I'll get an infection from the IV line." The remark drew smiles, but Dr. Casey still asked David for the required confirmation of his consent to the MAID procedure, to which he replied, "Yes."

Shortly before, David had asked to speak with Tim alone for a moment. "He asked me to make sure that he was dead after the procedure," Tim says. "His body was scheduled for cremation the next day. His worst fear was waking up as he was being cremated. So, after the MAID drugs were administered and the doctor noted the time of death, I sat with him for a further thirty minutes to ensure his final wish. It was all done just as he wanted it. Rational and methodical to the end, on his terms, reflecting in his death very much how he lived his life. It was perfect for him."

The obituary for David James Stephenson Hockey, edited and approved by David himself, included the line: "Our special thanks to Genevieve Casey and the MAID Network."

About four months after his father's MAID procedure, Tim's wife, Lana, was diagnosed with Stage 1(b) pancreatic cancer. What followed were many rounds of chemotherapy and then surgery. For a couple of years, the cancer seemed to be held at bay. Those were wonderful years, as Tim and Lana lived life to the fullest, knowing that pancreatic cancer had a habit of recurring.

In February 2024, Lana's worst fears were realized: the cancer had returned, this time in her bowel, causing intense pain. It was a terminal diagnosis, and her prognosis was "weeks to months." Chemotherapy would only extend her life to the latter end of that spectrum. Tim recalls, "Telling our two boys was the toughest part of the terminal diagnosis. A few days later, Lana started discussing MAID with me. She was very moved by how my dad had handled the end of his cancer journey, and she very much wanted something similar."

Lana, unlike the more reserved David, was gregarious and outgoing and would not go quietly. Tim explains, "She decided there would be no more chemo after a few rounds, that it wasn't worth it, that it stole her strength while giving her only a few more months. She wanted to be full-on Lana right to the end. Incidentally, she also had been intubated at one point previously with a breathing tube, and she told me in no uncertain terms, 'don't let them ever do that to me again.'" Tim took that message to heart.

Soon after sharing the news of her final diagnosis and her decision to opt for MAID, though not a specific date, one of her sons announced that he and his partner were planning an engagement party at the Hockey family home. At Lana's request, the engagement party was transformed into a wedding for seventy people in early March 2024, two weeks after Lana was released from the hospital. Lana believed that when you don't have much time left, you make the most of it.

To celebrate the newlyweds, Lana instructed Tim to buy them a house as a wedding gift. The initial plan was to find something affordable further from the city centre, but the urgency of the cancer and the looming deadline of the MAID procedure led Tim to buy a house just around the corner from their own home. Time was of the essence.

Three weeks after her son's wedding, as her strength began to wane, Lana celebrated her sixtieth birthday with a large party for friends and family. She had a particularly wide group of female companions dating back to her Ultimate Frisbee days, where she had also met Tim when they were both in their twenties. Her friends all knew about Lana's plan to pursue MAID. While they weren't told the exact date, they knew this gathering would be their last together. They created a wonderful book of memories, filled with text and pictures, that memorialized Lana's entire adult life. Lana was deeply moved by their effort and participation. She worked hard to ensure that her final terminal cancer journey would be life-affirming.

Similar to the memorial book, another group of friends, this one from outside Canada, created a quilt for Lana. Each panel commemorated their shared adventures, resulting in a beautiful memento of their time together. As I speak with Tim, the quilt rests on the couch in their home. It was this quilt, now a treasured heirloom, that Lana was wrapped in during her MAID procedure.

As the spring and early summer of 2024 progressed, Lana, aware of her dwindling time, devoted herself to completing other meaningful projects. For instance, she used an online service to record herself reading children's books, ensuring her future grandchildren could hear their grandmother's voice.

By August, Lana had grown very weak and was ready to say her final goodbyes. She and Tim hosted a large family barbecue on a Sunday. Lana presented everyone with a plain white T-shirt, then covered her hands and arms in paint. She embraced each family member, leaving her colourful handprints and armprints on their shirts as a lasting keepsake. Wearing the t-shirt would then be like receiving a hug from Lana. Her profound love for her family and her deeply human spirit shone brightly until the very end.

Interestingly, while Lana informed Tim and her sons that her MAID procedure would take place sometime in August, she withheld the specific date until just a few days prior. Tim's father, David, had taken a different approach, informing his family about a month in advance. Tim and Lana had discussed how this foreknowledge created a surreal sense of impending loss, something Lana hoped to avoid. Ultimately, even the inherent compassion within the MAID process cannot fully mask the deep emotional turmoil caused by someone's approaching death. MAID significantly reduces suffering, but cannot eliminate it entirely.

Two days after the family barbecue, Lana underwent her MAID procedure. She chose not to have her sons present in the room during the injection. She bid them tearful farewells at the door, and they left for their newly acquired house nearby. Tim stayed with Lana during the procedure, which unfolded peacefully, mirroring his father's experience four years prior.

Later that year, at Christmas, Tim and his two sons went to the storage room for the Christmas ornaments and other holiday decorations. As they began unpacking and decorating, Tim tried to maintain a cheerful atmosphere, but Lana's absence was palpable; she had always been the heart of their Christmas celebrations. Then, they opened the boxes and found a wonderful surprise: long, detailed notes from Lana to each of them. She gave instructions for everything, from which cousin received which gift, to virtual hugs and kisses. Thanks to MAID, Lana had been spared the intense stress, uncertainty, and pain of a natural death, allowing her to plan and organize her final days, and beyond, with purpose and meaning.

A year after Lana's MAID procedure, I spoke with Tim, asking how his perspective on her decision had changed with time.

"Cancer is terrible, and Lana's was particularly rough on her," he said. "But you have to play the cards life deals you, and Lana did that wonderfully. She was a planner all her life. It made so much sense to me, and to her, that she chose MAID."

As our conversation ended, I asked if he would consider MAID for himself, should the circumstances warrant it.

"I'm a planner, too," Tim replied.

At Lana's request, there was no obituary. However, she wrote the following message to her friends and family, which Tim emailed later the day she died:

From: Lana Hockey
Date: August 12, 2024 at 5:27:56 PM EDT
To: Tim Hockey [copied to friends/family]
Subject: A last goodbye . . .
"Somewhere over the rainbow . . ."

My dear friends,

As you know, for the past several months, I have been battling cancer . . . again. This note is my way of telling you that the fight is over, and the bad guy won.

Since receiving the terminal diagnosis in February, my life has been about checking things off a rather daunting to-do list and collecting joy. I'm happy to say that the list is done, and my joy bucket is overflowing.

Joy comes in many forms: from the in a lifetime joy of an impromptu wedding in our home; to the more simple joys of family dinners, card games around the kitchen table, walking around the neighbourhood holding hands with Tim, or drinking wine or eating cake (for breakfast!) while visiting with friends.

I'm grateful for all the memories you have shared of our adventures, and misadventures, over the years. Memories captured in the 60th birthday photo book so many contributed to; in the digital photo frame (some photos requiring explanation); in the knitted quilt that travelled the World to get here; in the texts, e-mails and WhatsApp messages. SO many memories . . . smiles triumphing over tears . . . so much love and support. There is a gift in knowing that your time is limited. Every moment becomes more precious . . . every word spoken, more meaningful.

Mostly, I'm grateful for having you in my life. Going through this last stage has taught me how very blessed I am to have an amazing, loving, devoted family and an awesome group of friends from all over the world.

Thank you for the part you played in my life story. It was a good one!

Life is short. Live Loud.

Love,

Lana

March 19, 1964 – August 12, 2024

". . . that's where you'll find me!"

In a more recent example, on February 20, 2026, *The Globe and Mail* published an obituary for Nadia Potts, who for two decades was a widely celebrated principal ballerina for the National Ballet of Canada. The obituary reported that Ms. Potts was diagnosed with ovarian cancer in 2022 and that on February 2, 2026, at age seventy-seven, she had MAID.

Eventually, you will experience the suffering inherent in your own dying process. If that process causes you intolerable suffering, in Canada you have the choice of ending that suffering through a dignified, compassionate, and merciful MAID provision, so long as you meet the criteria discussed in Chapter 3.

## Scenario 2: Avoiding Further Suffering from a Stroke or Accident

A stroke occurs when blood flow to the brain is interrupted, either by a haemorrhage or a blood clot that forms in or travels to the brain's arteries. This blockage deprives the brain of oxygen, causing damage that results in a stroke.

In Canada, between 62,000 and 108,000 people experience a stroke each year. The severity of a stroke depends on the extent of brain cell damage. Stroke is the third leading cause of death in Canada (13,833 deaths in 2023), following cancer (86,647) and heart disease (57,994), and is fatal for approximately 20 percent of those who experience one.

Stroke-related brain damage can impair mental and physical abilities. As many as 50 percent of stroke survivors require assistance with activities of daily living, such as getting out of bed or a chair, walking, using the toilet, eating, bathing, grooming, and dressing. Stroke can also affect independent living skills, including shopping, cooking, housekeeping, laundry, medication management, phone use, independent travel, and financial management.

Stroke survivors may also experience more subtle deficits, such as memory problems, depression, and fatigue. According to Heart and Stroke Canada, aphasia, which affects the ability to speak and understand language, affects one-third of stroke survivors. Depression occurs in one-third to one-half of stroke survivors. Cognitive abilities can also be affected.

The risk of stroke increases with age, with 80 percent of strokes occurring in people over sixty. Elderly Canadians who experience strokes often have other underlying medical conditions. For example, people with congenital heart disease are twice as likely to have a stroke.

Symptoms are typically most severe immediately after the stroke. Following a minor stroke, or a transient ischemic attack (TIA), often called a "mini-stroke," individuals can regain most or all of their pre-stroke abilities within days or weeks. Senator Murray Sinclair's recovery story, available on the Heart and Stroke website, is one such example.

A major stroke can leave you completely immobilized in the days following the event. With rigorous therapy, you will typically regain some function in speech, movement, and cognition. Maximum recovery is usually achieved within six months. The degree of impairment remaining at that point often becomes permanent.

Depending on your age, you may find your level of recovery and resulting quality of life unsatisfactory, particularly regarding your ability to perform daily and independent living activities. The extent of this permanent decline may lead you to consider MAID. Before MAID was legal in Canada, accepting this suffering was your only option. Now, if your post-stroke condition results in significant decline and intolerable suffering, you can choose to end your life with compassion through MAID, provided the stroke has not impaired your mental capacity to consent.

It is important to note that over 50 percent of stroke survivors experience cognitive impairment, ranging from 20 percent to 80 percent, within the first year. These impairments can affect reasoning and communication, which are critical for making informed medical decisions, including those about MAID. Furthermore, one-third of stroke survivors develop dementia within five years (though it can occur as early as one year), potentially triggered by the stroke itself. However, 40 percent of stroke survivors experience cognitive impairment that does not reach the level of dementia. Therefore, your ability to consent to medical treatment or MAID will depend on the degree of cognitive impairment you experience after your stroke.

In Canada, if you are a stroke survivor who continues to experience a significant decline from your pre-stroke life after your recovery period, and you suffer intolerably from stroke-related symptoms, you may be eligible for MAID. However, you must be able to consent. Be vigilant about how the stroke may diminish your mental capacity to consent over time. Assuming you retain sufficient capacity, MAID may be an option if you meet the criteria discussed in Chapter 3.

## Scenario 3: Avoiding Further Suffering from a Neurodegenerative Disease

Several diseases are classified as "neurodegenerative" because they involve the progressive loss of neurons, or nerve cells, which are the fundamental working units of the brain, spinal cord, and nerves. These diseases include Parkinson's (affecting approximately 110,000 people in Canada), Huntington's (7,000), Amyotrophic Lateral Sclerosis (ALS) (3,500), and Multiple Sclerosis (MS) (92,000). Dementia, including Alzheimer's disease, is also a neurodegenerative disease, but it will be addressed separately in Scenario 4 due to its specific impact on cognitive function.

Neurodegenerative diseases often share common symptoms, notably muscle weakness and loss of muscle control, frequently preceded by tremors and slow movement. These diseases are typically progressive, meaning symptoms worsen over time, leading to an irreversible decline in the ability to perform activities of daily living and, eventually, activities of independent living (as previously defined). The rate of decline can vary.

Prior to the introduction of MAID, the typical trajectory for individuals with neurodegenerative diseases often involved transitioning to a nursing home or similar facility when family caregivers could no longer manage their care. Currently, an estimated 170,000 individuals with neurodegenerative conditions reside in care homes across Canada.

While some individuals with advanced neurodegenerative disease may accept their condition and choose to reside in a care home contentedly, others may view this prospect with reluctance. Each person's experience with a neurodegenerative condition is unique, and their attitude toward the disease and its symptoms will vary accordingly.

If you have a neurodegenerative disease and find your condition unacceptable and your suffering intolerable, MAID may be an option, provided you have the capacity to consent and meet the other eligibility criteria outlined in Chapter 3. Although most neurodegenerative diseases eventually affect cognitive capacity in their later stages of irreversible decline, capacity is typically not compromised during much of the disease progression. However, individual circumstances vary, and it is essential to consult with a MAID provider to establish and monitor your specific situation.

If you have a neurodegenerative disease such as Parkinson's, Huntington's, ALS, or Multiple Sclerosis, and your suffering is intolerable, MAID is an option if you have the mental capacity to consent and meet the criteria outlined in Chapter 3. You would typically (but not necessarily) be considered for Track 2 MAID, which requires a ninety-day waiting period between the initial assessment and the provision of MAID. During this time, your MAID provider will discuss alternatives with you (as detailed in Chapter 3). Therefore, if you are considering Track 2 MAID for a neurodegenerative disease, factor in an additional three months, especially if your mental capacity is declining.

## Scenario 4: Avoiding Further Suffering from Dementia or Alzheimer's

Dementia is a cluster of symptoms that impairs memory and cognitive abilities, often accompanied by personality changes. It essentially diminishes brain function, leaving physical functions intact while the brain deteriorates. The daily impact of dementia can be devastating. You may lose the ability to engage in simple activities, such as playing games or preparing meals, due to memory loss. This decline can be particularly distressing, given the brain's central role in psychological and emotional well-being.

As the disease progresses, other common behaviours may emerge. Spatial awareness deteriorates, making it impossible to navigate familiar routes. Sleep patterns become erratic, and repetitive, nonsensical behaviours may develop. Eventually, the burden of care becomes too great for one person, often leading to placement in a care home (over half of Canadians in institutional care have dementia). Ironically, individuals with dementia are often unaware of their condition, making it difficult to reassure them when they become agitated by memory loss. In institutional care, autonomy is invariably lost, potentially leading to paranoia. Restraints, both physical and chemical, are sometimes used to manage dementia patients in such settings.

An estimated 770,000 Canadians live with some form of dementia, with approximately 62,500 new cases diagnosed each year. Alzheimer's disease accounts for 60 percent of these cases. Other significant causes of dementia include Lewy body dementia (caused by protein clumps), vascular dementia (resulting from blood flow issues like strokes), and frontotemporal dementia (due to damage to the frontal lobe of the brain). The following discussion will primarily focus on Alzheimer's disease due to its prevalence.

**Important Note:** The following descriptions, including symptoms and timelines, are general composites based on various sources. While they aim to represent a "typical" disease progression, individual experiences can vary significantly. If you suspect you have dementia (or Alzheimer's, etc.), consulting with healthcare professionals for a proper assessment is crucial.

A "typical" case of Alzheimer's disease (as described earlier) involves a roughly ten-year progressive decline in memory and cognitive function, unfolding in the following stages:

- Mild Alzheimer's (diagnosis to twelve to eighteen months): characterized by impaired judgment; increasing difficulty recalling words and recent conversations; repetitive questioning; spatial disorientation; challenges with problem-solving and organization; mood swings, increased anxiety, and agitation leading to social withdrawal; suspicion, confusion, and early paranoia.
- Moderate Alzheimer's (nineteen months to six years): progression to forgetting the purpose of familiar objects (e.g., car keys); mixing up objects (e.g., flushing garbage down the toilet); inability to manage "executive functions" like finances; complete social withdrawal; and, typically between two and three years post-diagnosis, an inability to recognize family members.
- Severe Alzheimer's (seven to ten years): often requiring care in a specialized facility due to an inability to respond to the environment. This stage involves an inability to hold a conversation; frequent and severe agitation and aggression, often accompanied by psychosis; risk of self-harm; the need for a secure environment to prevent wandering; and, in the final three months, a significant reduction in verbal communication (e.g., uttering only six words a day), difficulty swallowing, and incontinence.

It is important to remember that these timelines are approximate, and individual experiences with dementia will vary. Furthermore, the earlier description assumes prompt medical attention and diagnosis upon symptom onset. However, it is estimated that one-third of dementia/ Alzheimer's patients never receive an official diagnosis, often due to fear of the diagnosis and its implications.

Your brain arguably defines who you are. Therefore, dementia can fundamentally alter your identity, transforming you into someone unrecognizable compared to your former self. In Canada, MAID offers a choice: to allow the disease to progress and become a different person, or to end your life while you still retain your essential self.

Currently, as explained in Chapter 5 (see section on Advance Requests), Canadian law does not allow individuals with Alzheimer's to make Advance Requests for MAID to be administered at a future point when they have lost capacity. Even in Quebec, where advance requests are permitted, it's uncertain whether a MAID provider will honour a request made in advance (again, see Chapter 5).

Consequently, after an Alzheimer's diagnosis, once you experience a significant decline and suffer intolerably, your only option for MAID is while you still possess sufficient mental capacity. For MAID eligibility, an "advanced state of irreversible decline in capability" due to dementia is defined as imminent loss of capacity. Practically, this means pursuing MAID while loss of capacity is imminent, but before it actually occurs. To ensure access to MAID for Alzheimer's, it's advisable to proceed relatively soon after imminent loss of capacity becomes apparent. This requires close communication with your MAID provider to monitor your capacity.

In 2023, 106 Canadians received MAID, citing dementia as their sole underlying condition; approximately three-quarters of these cases fell under Track 1, and the remainder under Track 2. In 2024, this number rose to 368. Presumably, these 474 individuals experienced the symptoms and decline discussed earlier in this section.

Recent press reports highlight Robert Munsch, the acclaimed children's author, as another individual choosing MAID to alleviate the suffering associated with Alzheimer's. Diagnosed with Alzheimer's and Parkinson's in 2021, his subsequent decline has been closely followed by journalists. As of April 2026, when this book went to press, reports indicated that he had lost the ability to recall words and was no longer able to write. Having been approved for MAID, Munsch has publicly stated his intention to pursue it once he can no longer communicate verbally. He is presumably working closely with a MAID provider to monitor his mental capacity, ensuring he retains the necessary cognitive function at the time of the procedure.

In contrast to Munsch's approach, facilitated by Canada's MAID system, consider Terry Pratchett, the UK's best-selling author of the 1990s, with over 100 million books sold in forty-three languages. Diagnosed with early-onset Alzheimer's in 2007 at age fifty-nine, he was unable to write dedications at book signings by 2008. Two years post-diagnosis, Pratchett expressed his desire for MAID in an article, an option unavailable in the UK then and now. Following his 2011 documentary on assisted death, *Terry Pratchett: Choosing to Die*, he stated, "It should be possible for someone stricken with a serious and ultimately fatal illness to choose to die peacefully with medical help, rather than suffer." He ultimately died from complications of Alzheimer's in 2015 at age sixty-six.

Further illustrating the complexities of dementia, consider an open letter posted on August 18, 2014, by Gillian Bennett (https://www.deadatnoon.com/), then eighty-five, on her website *deadatnoon.com*. Bennett ended her life that day due to her dementia. While her letter predates Canada's MAID legislation, it poignantly articulates the reasons why many Canadians with dementia find solace in the availability of MAID under appropriate circumstances. Bennett's letter also underscores the immense burden and loss of dignity associated with taking one's own life, a reality faced by many before MAID was available in Canada for individuals suffering intolerably from incurable medical conditions. Twelve years later, Canadians can find comfort, and perhaps pride, in having a legal MAID system that allows those suffering intolerably from a medical condition, including dementia/ Alzheimer's in suitable cases, to request medical assistance in dying with dignity and compassion.

> **August 18, 2014**—I will take my life today around noon. It is time. Dementia is taking its toll and I have nearly lost myself. I have nearly lost *me*. Jonathan [Jillian's husband], the straightest and brightest of men, will be at my side as a loving witness.
>
> I have known that I have dementia, a progressive loss of memory and judgment, for three years. It is a stealthy, stubborn and oh-so reliable disease. I might have preferred an exotic ailment whose name came trippingly off the tongue, but no, what I have is entirely typical. I find it a boring disease, and despite the sweetness and politeness of my family I am bright enough to be aware of how boring they find it, too. It is so rough on my husband, Jonathan. I don't think my lovely cat has noticed, but I'm not sure.
>
> Dementia gives no quarter and admits no bargaining. Research tells us that it's a "silent disease," one that can lurk for years or even decades before its symptoms become obvious. Ever so gradually at first, much faster now, I am turning into a vegetable. I find it hard to keep in my mind that my granddaughter is coming in three days' time and not today. "Where do we keep the X?" (coffee / milkshake-maker / backspace on my keyboard / the book I was just reading) happens

all the time. I have constantly to monitor what I say in an attempt not to make some gross error of judgment.

There comes a time, in the progress of dementia, when one is no longer competent to guide one's own affairs. I want out before the day when I can no longer assess my situation, or take action to bring my life to an end. There could also come a time when I simply must make a decision based on my deteriorating physical health. I do not like hospitals—they are dirty places. Any doctor will tell you to stay out of them if you possibly can. I would not want a fall, a stroke, or some unforeseen complication to mess up my decision to cost Canada as little as possible in my declining years.

Understand that I am giving up nothing that I want by committing suicide. All I lose is an indefinite number of years of being a vegetable in a hospital setting, eating up the country's money but having not the faintest idea of who I am.

Each of us is born uniquely and dies uniquely. I think of dying as a final adventure with a predictably abrupt end. I know when it's time to leave and I do not find it scary.

There are so many things we obsess about. We seem to have a need to get things right. Should we bring a bottle of wine or some flowers to the party? Will jeans and my new boots work or is that too casual? How do I find a new mate?

We do NOT talk much about how we die. Yet facing death is thoroughly interesting and absorbing and challenging. I have choices which I have reviewed, and either adopted or discarded. I think I have hit upon the right choice for me.

I have talked it over with friends and relatives. It is not a forbidden topic. Anything but.

Every day I lose bits of myself, and it's obvious that I am heading toward the state that all dementia patients eventually get to:

not knowing who I am and requiring full-time care. I know as I write these words that within six months or nine months or twelve months, I, Gillian, will no longer be here. What is to be done with my carcass? It will be physically alive but there will be no one inside.

I have done my homework. I have reviewed my options:

1. Have a minder care for my mindless body. This would involve financial hardship for those I leave behind, or involve them in a seemingly endless round of chores that could erode even their fondest memories of me.
2. Request whatever care the government is willing to provide. (The facility will expect my husband, children, grandchildren, to visit often to thank the caretakers for how well they are looking after the carcass. Fair enough, but not what I wish for my family.)
3. End my own life by taking adequate barbiturates to do the job before my mind has totally gone. Ethically, this seems to me the right thing to do.

I can live or vegetate for perhaps ten years in hospital at Canada's expense, costing anywhere from $50,000 to $75,000 per year. That is only the beginning of the damage. Nurses, who thought they were embarked on a career that had great meaning, find themselves perpetually changing my diapers and reporting on the physical changes of an empty husk. It is ludicrous, wasteful and unfair.

My family, all of whom are rational and funny to boot, would not visit me in hospital, because they know I would not want them to.

The world strains under the weight of an aging population. We are living longer, and our life expectancies continue to grow. By

2045, the ratio of working-age citizens to their elderly dependents will become increasingly burdensome in almost every part of the world. In Canada and the United States, the ratio is expected to be sixteen workers for every ten elderly dependents. It is a social and economic disaster in the making.

Yet most people say they would like to live to 90 or 100, or even beyond.

There are many ethical issues here: life extension radically alters people's ideas of what it is to be human—and not for the better. As we, the elderly, undergo manifold operations and become gaga while taking up a hospital bed, our grandchildren's schooling, their educational, athletic, and cultural opportunities, will be squeezed dry.

The heart of the problem is arithmetic: The post-World War II Social Welfare State, created at a moment when the baby boom was still gestating, is built on a generational Ponzi scheme. As life expectancy increases and birth rates decline, the population pyramid is being inverted—and in some countries that is causing the entire economy to topple.

Everybody by the age of 50 who is mentally competent should make a Living Will that states how she wants to die, the circumstances under which she does not want to be resuscitated, etc. Add a statement such as: "If I am ill and frail and have an infection such as pneumonia, do not attempt to restore me to life with antibiotics. Pray let me pass. I do not give any relatives or doctors or psychiatrists the right to squelch this decision." One's general practitioner would have a copy.

Legally, everyone should have an obligation to make a Will, which would be stored electronically, could not be destroyed, and would be available automatically to any hospital in the world.

What about a person who refuses to make a Will? There should be a fallback Will that applies to everyone who has not done his civic duty. I do not have all the answers, but I do think I'm raising questions that need to be raised.

Three outsize institutions: the medical profession, the law, and the church will challenge and fight any transformative change. Yet we all hear of changes in each of these professions that suggest a broader approach, guided and informed by empathy. My hope is that all of these institutions will continue to transform themselves, and that the medical profession will mandate, through sensitive and appropriate protocols, the administration of a lethal dose to end the suffering of a terminally ill patient, in accordance with her Living Will.

Life seems somewhat like a party that I was dropped into. At first I was shy and awkward and didn't know what the rules were. I was afraid of doing the wrong thing. It turned out that I was there to enjoy myself and I didn't know how to do that. Someone kind talked to me and made me laugh. I began to understand that actually I had to make up my own rules and then live by them.

I did pick up that I needed to know when to leave, and that is now.

All members of my immediate family are in Vancouver: daughter, son, two granddaughters and four grandsons. All know that it matters to me not to become a burden to them, or to Canada. I have discussed my situation with them all. In our family it is recognized that any adult has the right to make her own decision.

Just in case anyone is tempted to think I must be brave to off myself, you should know that I am a big sookie. I am sorely fearful of being alone in the dark. I am scared something will get me. I do not want to die alone. If my cat were failing in the way that I am,

I would mix some sleeping medication in with top-quality ground beef, and when she fell asleep, carry her lovingly to the garden and do the rest. Who wants to die surrounded by strangers, no matter how excellent their care and competence?

I have had a husband beyond compare, and children and grandchildren who have outstripped me in most meaningful ways. Since I was seven I have had wonderful friends, whom I did and still do adore.

This is all much tougher than it need be on Jonathan, and I wish he did not have to be alone with his wife's corpse. Canadian law makes it a crime for anyone to assist a person committing suicide, and Jonathan, therefore, will in no way assist me. Our children, Sara and Guy, would so willingly be with their father, but the laws being what they are, we will not put them in jeopardy.

Today, now, I go cheerfully and so thankfully into that good night. Jonathan, the courageous, the faithful, the true and the gentle, surrounds me with company. I need no more.

It is almost noon.

Consider, for another more recent example involving dementia, an obituary that notes the deceased began exhibiting signs of Alzheimer's in 2022 and subsequently lost all memory. The obituary expresses gratitude that the deceased suffered for "only" three years. It would be insightful to know if the deceased, while still capable, considered MAID to avoid what seems to have been a challenging disease progression. This scenario echoes President Ronald Reagan's experience with Alzheimer's. On November 5, 1994, the former president released a letter announcing his diagnosis, writing, in part: "I only wish there was some way I could spare Nancy [Reagan's wife] from this painful experience." Because MAID was unavailable in the United States at the time, President Reagan lived with Alzheimer's for ten more years, until his death on June 5, 2004. Even today, MAID is not an option for dementia patients in the United States. Fortunately, in Canada, MAID allows individuals to exercise autonomy and choice regarding dementia, Alzheimer's, and similar conditions, provided they carefully manage the MAID process in consultation with a MAID provider.

A recent obituary in *The Globe and Mail* ("Diplomat Helped Canada Win a Seat on the UN Security Council, December 6, 2025") provides a compelling example of a Canadian exercising this choice. The obituary recounts the story of David M. Malone, a distinguished Canadian diplomat and former United Nations Under-Secretary-General. After being diagnosed with Alzheimer's disease and experiencing memory loss, Mr. Malone, aged seventy-one, chose to end his life through MAID rather than endure years of cognitive decline. The day before his death, he attended a concert featuring Copland's *Appalachian Spring*, and the night before, he enjoyed dinner with a close friend. He passed away with five people at his bedside. The *Globe* article quotes Mr. Malone's long-time friend, Shashi Tharoor, who initially tried to dissuade him from MAID but later understood his reasoning: "David asserted a final act of agency. He refused to let disease dictate the terms of his existence. He chose to leave while he was still himself. In doing so, he left his friends not with the image of a man diminished, but with the memory of a person who remained brilliant, humane and generous to the last."

In Canada, MAID offers individuals suffering intolerably from Alzheimer's or other dementia-inducing illnesses the option to end their lives with dignity, compassion, and peace before the disease entirely deprives them of decision-making capacity. However, careful timing of the final decision is crucial. If the decision is delayed until the individual has progressed into an irreversible state of cognitive decline and is no longer able to consent to MAID, they will be required to continue suffering, potentially for years (again, see aforementioned "Important Note" regarding timelines). An exception exists in Quebec, where individuals can complete an Advance Request for MAID while they still possess the capacity to do so (the Quebec Advance Request is described in Chapter 5 under the section on Advance Requests; it is not, however, a perfect solution, as noted in Chapter 5).

## CHAPTER 2

# HELPING LOVED ONES THROUGH MAID

This chapter addresses those who have elected to undergo MAID, as well as family members or close friends of someone who has made this choice. Facing this situation often raises novel personal issues and affects family dynamics. Of course, any impending death, including a natural one, presents challenges to the person nearing the end of life and their loved ones. For instance, any adult with assets should complete and sign a will, the legal document that dictates how property is to be distributed among family members, charities, and other beneficiaries upon death. You may also decide how your remains are to be handled, whether through burial, cremation, or other methods like composting (through terramation).

However, MAID differs from natural death in significant ways, requiring you and those helping you through the MAID process to consider unique issues. This chapter explores some of the more important ones. Keep in mind that in Canada, only about 16,500 people (16,499 in 2024) undergo MAID each year, while approximately 330,000 die "traditionally." If you choose MAID, you will likely be the first in your family to do so, and most, if not all, of your family members and close friends will also be directly exposed to MAID for the first time through your experience.

## Why Talk about MAID?

Perhaps your most significant challenge is simply communicating with family and friends about MAID in a meaningful and respectful manner. This assumes, however, that you wish to discuss your decision with them. You could choose to undergo MAID without informing anyone. You are not obligated to share your MAID journey. Or, you may not have family with whom to discuss it. Everyone's life is different, including yours.

However, if you have family and are inclined to exclude them from your MAID decision, consider reconsidering. Even if you believe the decision is solely yours—and it is—consider the impact on those in your family. You are, in effect, making a decision that will influence your legacy, or at least how people perceive you and your legacy after you are gone. If familial relationships have deteriorated over time, now might be the time to reconnect and strive for some level of understanding while there is still time.

Talking about your impending death, and MAID (if you're considering it), can be beneficial. Research suggests that discussing end-of-life issues with even just a few people can reduce psychological stress. Reflecting on your life and discussing your death can ultimately help you find peace, achieve a sense of completion, and make sense of your life's meaning. This process can also help you live more fully in the present moment, fostering a sense of calm and reducing the fear or dread associated with death. Consequently, you may live the remainder of your life with greater purpose and peace—a worthwhile outcome if MAID helps you reach this state.

## How to Talk about MAID

Discussions about MAID can be challenging, as individuals, including loved ones, may hold differing views on this serious topic. Furthermore, before discussing MAID, you might need to explain for the first time that you have a terminal illness causing severe suffering or that your chronic condition has become intolerable. This initial information can be overwhelming, even before introducing the subject of MAID itself. It's important to recognize that the person you're speaking with needs time to process a significant amount of new information.

Here are some suggestions to facilitate your MAID discussions:

- Difficult conversations often require time: avoid expecting someone to change their mind or support your decision after a single discussion; the initial conversation might simply involve expressing your views and listening to theirs.
- Frame it as a discussion: "Would you be open to hearing my thoughts about MAID?"; keep the tone relatively low-key; "Here's what others have said about MAID"; avoid being overly persuasive.
- Use open-ended questions: "How familiar are you with MAID?"; "What questions do you have about it?"; you are likely well-informed about MAID, while others may not be, which is another reason to initiate these discussions sooner rather than later.

If you are in the pre-MAID procedure phase (i.e., you have already been assessed as eligible), you may feel pressured as your time is running short. While your inclination might be to avoid discussions, resist that urge. The person you're speaking with is someone you love or a good friend, so make time for them. They will have their own perspectives, and allowing their last experience with you to be civil will be meaningful for them. Ideally, they will reciprocate with a similar approach. Civility should be the guiding principle for everyone. Remember, the purpose of this discussion, including listening to them, isn't to change their mind but to explain your decision.

Focus on why you believe what you believe, and avoid excessive criticism of their views. Changing someone's mind in a single conversation is unlikely; speak from the heart and explain your reasoning. Your hope is that later, when they reflect on your discussion, they will become more understanding, even if only partially. Keep in mind that people need time to process and adjust their perspectives.

Correct any misinformation they have. Ask them about their thoughts and what they believe to be the relevant facts. There is a lot of inaccurate information about MAID circulating, particularly on social media. Understand their factual basis and then address any misunderstandings calmly and reasonably.

Sometimes, you must agree to disagree. On a topic like MAID, some people will simply hold different views. For example, they might approach MAID from a religious perspective. In these cases, you may need to adjust your objective. While you may desire a respectful dialogue, they might never support your plans for MAID. This is unavoidable sometimes, and you may need to move on, as you likely have other MAID-related conversations to have.

## When to Start Talking about MAID

To build consensus within your family about MAID, it's helpful to start the conversation sooner rather than later, perhaps including one or two close friends. Given that approximately 37 percent of MAID recipients in Canada are between fifty-five and seventy-four, consider researching

MAID in your mid-fifties and discussing it with your spouse or adult children, even in general terms. Initiating a discussion about MAID with your family doctor around this time is also a good idea. It's beneficial for these individuals to understand your feelings about MAID, and for you to understand their perspectives as well.

You might first start thinking about MAID after an initial engagement with the healthcare system for a serious, but soon resolved, medical issue. For example, a minor heart attack might lead to a stent insertion to relieve an arterial blockage, an almost routine procedure in many urban hospitals nowadays. While recovering in your room for a day or two, you might ask your attending physician some high-level questions about MAID, perhaps about their general experience with it in the hospital, or with patients suffering from end-stage congenital heart failure. Nothing too detailed, but enough to start a dialogue that you can then continue with others in the healthcare system as needed.

## Your Lead Supporter

Years pass, perhaps even a decade or two, and you now face a dire and incurable medical condition, a serious decline, and intolerable suffering. After weeks of contemplation, you decide to choose MAID. Before addressing specific MAID issues, consider the people, or likely the single person, who will help you manage the process. This typically will be your spouse, if you have one; otherwise, an adult child; or, if you have no children, your best friend. Let's call this person your "lead supporter."

Ideally, a lead supporter would help you through a natural death as well, but there is one major difference with MAID. With a natural death, your lead supporter will likely not question the way you die; the dying process tends to have its own internal "logic" (though they may question particular steps along the way, such as whether, and when, to stop a particular treatment). With MAID, it's important that your lead supporter, who will be closely at your side, either agrees with your decision or at least supports it, even if they have personal reservations. The dying process is emotional enough as it is. It is much harder if the person closest to you throughout this novel exercise constantly questions your decision.

Therefore, before choosing a lead supporter, have a serious discussion with them about MAID. Essentially, ask them what they think about it, and about your plan to access it. Be frank; it will be helpful to have someone in this position you trust and who is a comfort to you. If they hesitate, consider another family member or friend. Remember, the MAID process will be more challenging if your core support group is fragmented.

If you previously signed a Power of Attorney for Personal Care, review it to confirm who you appointed to make medical decisions on your behalf should you become incapacitated. Ideally, this person should also be your lead supporter for MAID, as conflicts could arise if different individuals are responsible for these crucial medical decisions. If you choose a different lead supporter for MAID, consider also appointing them as your power of attorney for personal care, ensuring they can make medical decisions if you lose capacity. Taking these steps will help streamline your MAID journey. (It's important to note that while a power of attorney can make other medical decisions, actual MAID decisions cannot be delegated.)

## The Timing of Your MAID

A key difference between a natural death and MAID is the ability to set a specific date and time for the MAID procedure. This presents both opportunities and responsibilities that you should address. Alternatively, your lead supporter can manage these aspects on your behalf, but only after you have established your overall preferences.

MAID allows family and friends from afar to plan visits before your passing. However, this ability to plan may also create sensitivities with estranged or distant relatives. With MAID, there is a greater expectation of inclusivity in pre-MAID ceremonies. The common excuse for natural deaths—"Oh, Leslie died suddenly"—no longer applies if you choose MAID. For example, your lead supporter can't use the unexpected timing of death to justify excluding relatives from your MAID celebration of life (discussed below). While you may still choose to exclude someone, the timing of your death will no longer serve as a convenient justification.

Another significant difference is that family and friends typically don't question the timing of a natural death, as it's seen as beyond anyone's control. However, with MAID, you have some control over your departure date (though not always, especially if you postpone your MAID provision until late in the dying process). Should you delay your MAID provision until after a grandchild's birthday or your wedding anniversary? These considerations are less relevant with a natural death, which typically occurs when it occurs, and is generally accepted by all.

For instance, Lana Hockey in Chapter 1 extended her MAID provision to attend her son's wedding. This illustrates the types of accommodations possible with MAID. However, be mindful that as your MAID date approaches, your strength and stamina may decrease, and palliative care medications could cause side effects. Consequently, avoid being overly ambitious with your plans simply because you are undergoing MAID.

## When to Share the Proposed MAID Date

Imagine it is March, and you have been approved for MAID. Given the progression of your end-stage cancer and increasing pain, you anticipate being ready for MAID in June, three months away. Should you immediately share a specific June date with family and friends? This decision requires careful consideration, as providing a precise date so far in advance can create unease. The specificity might make your impending death weigh heavily on them for an extended period.

Consider indicating a more general timeframe, such as "late June" or "late spring," allowing people to be available and out-of-towners to plan visits. However, if you plan a pre-MAID celebration of life (see following text), aim to give people a couple of months' notice to mark their calendars. These types of questions require careful thought with MAID.

## New MAID Rituals

Since the dawn of humanity, death, dying, and their associated rituals have been central concerns. Ancient civilizations in Egypt, China, Greece, India, and Rome all grappled with how we die, the meaning of death, and the proper conduct of the dying process. With contemporary philosophy, morals, and the advancements of modern medicine, we need to update our rituals for the dying process.

In some communities, it's increasingly common for surviving spouses or children to host a "celebration of life" months after a loved one's death.

This can be a wonderful event, allowing attendance from friends and acquaintances who couldn't make the funeral. Typically uplifting, these gatherings feature touching tributes, often with humour, which helps attendees process their grief.

The primary drawback of a celebration of life held after a natural death is the absence of the deceased. I recall attending such a gathering for a dear high school friend several years ago, and it was profoundly moving. Speaker after speaker recounted how Sal (not his real name) had touched their lives, expressing deep respect and admiration. I learned so much about him that day. As the eulogies concluded, tears streaming down my face, I turned to my wife, also tearful, and remarked, "This was very moving, but it's too bad that Sal wasn't here. He would have loved it." Instead, all that was present was a large photograph of Sal at the front of the hall.

However, with MAID, you have the option of attending your own celebration of life by holding the event *before* the procedure. You can listen and, depending on your condition, even speak, allowing for personal goodbyes. Your presence can make the experience all the more meaningful, with the MAID provision scheduled for the days that follow.

Of course, a pre-MAID celebration of life isn't for everyone. It's simply another choice made possible by MAID, but by no means a requirement. Some may prefer a party or an intimate gathering, while others may wish for a quiet departure. MAID is about empowering and supporting individual choices.

If you do choose to have a celebration of life, keep in mind that MAID may be a new concept for those attending. The idea of a pre-MAID celebration might feel strange or even unsettling to them. They may question whether it's appropriate for their children or, if religious, have concerns about the event given the impending MAID procedure. How can you address these concerns?

In the invitation, be clear about your intentions: that this is a celebration of life preceding MAID. Consider including a paragraph explaining your reasons for choosing MAID. This isn't about justifying your decision, but rather providing context to your extended family and friends, ensuring they feel informed. After all, they care about you and will want to understand your perspective.

Ideally, the people you invite to your celebration of life will see it as a chance to share memories and support each other in light of your impending death. This ceremony can help people begin grieving while also honouring a life well-lived. Expect both tears and laughter, as both can help you and your guests cope with your end-of-life situation or chronic medical condition, as well as your decision to pursue MAID.

## It's All about Communication

When introducing the idea of a MAID ritual to family and friends, open discussions are key. For friends, consider including a detailed explanation with the invitation to your celebration of life. This doesn't need to be lengthy, but it should address why you've chosen MAID and what it involves. While some friends may decline after reading this, those who attend will appreciate the advance notice.

If friends decline, you or your lead supporter (keeping in mind you may be experiencing significant fatigue) can try to speak with them individually. Ultimately, it's their decision to understand and accept your choice regarding MAID; you shouldn't feel pressured to change your mind based on their beliefs. Should they face similar suffering from a debilitating dying process or chronic disease (in the case of Track 2 MAID), they can then decide their own path. For now, you've made your decision, and hopefully, they will respect it, regardless of how unfamiliar or uncomfortable it may be.

With close family members, especially a spouse and adult children, it's best to begin discussing your MAID intentions early. Discovering a parent's decision to pursue MAID just ten days before the procedure can be shocking and create lasting tension, potentially clouding the memories of surviving loved ones. To the extent possible, try to avoid this outcome, particularly if you consider bringing family members closer together to be part of your legacy.

To achieve this goal, the more time you allow your loved ones to process your MAID decision, the better. Ideally, begin this process well before your medical condition significantly deteriorates. You may have been contemplating MAID for some time, and your loved ones will need time to catch up. While this is not an easy conversation, starting the discussion as early as reasonably possible can be beneficial.

## Pre-Diagnosis MAID Discussions

As previously mentioned, if you are considering MAID after receiving a difficult medical diagnosis, an early discussion with your loved ones, especially your lead supporter, is advisable. However, you can take this a step further.

If you are in your early to mid-sixties (or even late fifties), in good health, but inclined toward choosing MAID if you were to encounter certain medical conditions, it can be wise to initiate a discussion about your intentions with your spouse and adult children. Indeed, airing your views on MAID before the added pressure of a specific, life-altering medical diagnosis can be useful. This allows for questions about your inclination toward MAID to be addressed in a relaxed setting. Furthermore, your family will be reassured, knowing that a later decision to pursue MAID was not a sudden shift, but rather a continuation of your previously expressed views.

Similarly, if you are an adult child in your mid-to-late thirties and your parents in their sixties have not broached the topic of MAID, you might consider initiating the conversation. Again, without a specific medical diagnosis looming, a discussion around the dinner table may flow more easily. This may also involve basic information sharing if they haven't previously considered MAID.

## If You're a Family Member

Imagine you are an adult child, and your parent has just announced their decision to end their suffering through MAID. This news is unexpected, especially because you believed they were managing their chronic or other medical condition effectively. You had arranged a tour of a care home, ensured the wheelchair was provided, and thought everything was progressing smoothly. You anticipated your parent having another ten to fifteen years of life. Now, your parent informs you that they will undergo MAID in two months.

What can you do? First, simply listen. Really listen to what your mom or dad is saying. They are not only conveying information, but hoping for alignment, or at least for your support. You mean the world to them, and they've thought a lot about this moment. They want you to agree with, or at least support, their decision.

If you agree with their MAID decision, then your response is presumably simple: "Of course, Dad, I totally get it, and I will support you in any way that I can." However, if you have any hesitation, concerns, or simply don't agree with MAID, please show your father or mother empathy. They have given this a lot of thought, and this is one of the biggest decisions they will ever make. It will be difficult for them if you push back and withhold approval. Announcing "I don't agree with what you are doing, and I will not be a part of your plan to commit suicide," or words to that effect, will devastate them. What end, precisely, do you think these words will achieve? They are not really asking permission, though they would prefer to have your approval or blessing. Whatever you do, try not to get angry. You might feel strong emotions, including anger, but consider how your actions will affect your relationship with your mom or dad.

If you don't agree with MAID in principle, you're of course entitled to your own views and opinions. When you reach the stage in life where your parent is, you'll be free to decide how you wish to proceed. But facing their decision, this is not about you; it's about your mom or dad. What they deserve, and what you should give them, is at least the following: "Dad/Mom, I'm so sorry to hear you're suffering so much. I don't know exactly what I think about MAID, but frankly that's not the point. What is important is that you have made this decision, and I'll support you all the way to the end. I love you."

Then, when you are witnessing your parent lying on a bed about to undergo MAID, something like the following would be good: "Dad/Mom, I'm going to miss you, and I see now how this decision to have MAID was so right for you. I love you." This will be their last thought as they leave the world. Thank you—well done.

## Accepting Your Friend's MAID Decision

Similarly, here's some advice for when a friend informs you of their decision to pursue MAID. If you support their choice, express your agreement. More importantly, if you disagree—whether due to religious beliefs or differing personal values, especially in cases of Track 2 MAID where a chronic condition causes suffering—please keep those views to yourself. This sensitive situation is not about you. You are free to make your own choices when faced with a similar situation. For now, your role is to support your friend and their primary caregiver during this difficult time. If you cannot offer supportive or helpful words, it's best to remain silent.

If you have reservations about MAID but are invited to your friend's pre-MAID celebration of life, and are encouraged to bring family, including children, attend and keep your doubts private. Focus on your relationship with your friend, who is offering a heartfelt opportunity to say goodbye. Embrace it. If your children have questions, answer them honestly and neutrally. Frame it as, "It's wonderful we live in a free society where everyone gets to decide how they want their life to end if they have a medical condition causing them intolerable suffering." You can share your personal views, ideally without judgment, and reveal your preferences if asked. However, allow your children to form their own opinions, or at least understand that they will have the freedom to do so when the time comes.

What if you belong to a religion that forbids MAID for its members? As discussed in Chapter 5, while Catholic Church leaders remain opposed to MAID, other Christian denominations, such as the United Church and Anglicans, are showing flexibility, as are many Catholic followers. Similarly, within the Jewish community, while some firmly oppose MAID, others, including members and leaders, support congregants who choose it. As noted in Chapter 5, times are changing.

This can be challenging. Recently, a Christian minister's spouse chose MAID. The minister supported their spouse throughout the process but struggled with whether to be fully truthful with their faith community.

Ultimately, some people of faith will understand and accept the decision to pursue MAID, while others will not. Presumably, over time, the former group will grow, and the latter will diminish.

## Grieving and MAID

Regardless of how you die, whether naturally or through MAID, your family and close friends will grieve your loss. They will experience deep sadness and feel bereft, and bereavement is never easy.

However, as you consider your path and options, take comfort in knowing that your family and friends may find solace in your choice of MAID. It demonstrates your control over the dying process or the suffering caused by your debilitating chronic condition. They will remember that you avoided the worst suffering that often precedes death, or that you shortened the intolerable suffering from your condition. While this will not diminish their profound loss, your decision will bring them some peace during a difficult time. MAID can reduce not only your suffering, but also soothe the grief of your loved ones.

## MAID without Loved Ones

The preceding discussion assumes you will involve loved ones in your MAID journey. If you live alone and have no family or friends you wish to include, support is still available. Two groups, MFSS and Bridge C-14, offer MAID volunteers to support people considering MAID. Their contact information is at the end of Chapter 3. If you live in Toronto or Victoria, BC, consider MAiDHouse, which provides a safe space for MAID procedures. Their contact information is at the end of Chapter 7.

Some individuals who choose MAID, despite having family and friends, prefer not to involve them, believing "my MAID is none of their business." As mentioned, you are not obligated to discuss your decision with anyone. However, reaching out to even one or two loved ones may improve your pre-MAID experience and the legacy you leave behind (assuming they eventually learn of your decision). The weeks or months before death can be difficult, but also meaningful, offering opportunities for reflection, deep thought, understanding, and perhaps even inner peace. Many find that connecting with family and friends, even after a recent reconciliation, can enrich these experiences. Ultimately, however, the decision is yours.

## CHAPTER 3

# THE BASICS OF CANADIAN MAID

In Canada, if you have a serious and incurable medical condition that has caused an advanced, irreversible decline in your capabilities, resulting in intolerable suffering, and if you meet certain other criteria and safeguards, you have the option to request MAID. If you choose to do so, a MAID provider (either a doctor or a nurse practitioner) can end your life with dignity, empathy, and compassion. This chapter outlines the practical *criteria* you must meet to be eligible for MAID and describes *the MAID process* itself, from the initial eligibility assessment to the administration of medications.

If you have recently received a medical diagnosis that makes you wonder about your future, or if your chronic medical condition has worsened, you likely have questions about how MAID works. This chapter is intended to help you consider MAID, but you will need to speak with a MAID provider to understand how it might apply to your specific situation. To that end, information on how to contact a MAID provider in your province is provided at the end of this chapter.

## The Basics of MAID

To receive MAID in Canada, you must meet certain medical criteria, administrative requirements, and safeguards. These are briefly outlined here and discussed in more detail later in this chapter. To be eligible for MAID, you must:

- have a serious and incurable illness, disease, or disability;
- be in an advanced state of irreversible decline in capability; and
- be suffering intolerably from the medical condition or the decline in capability, and this suffering cannot be relieved.

In addition, to access MAID you must:

- be eighteen years of age or older; and
- be eligible for public healthcare in the Canadian province where you reside.

Finally, to access MAID you must:

- have made a voluntary request for MAID that was not the result of external pressure;
- have sufficient mental capacity to give informed consent;
- have given consent to MAID after being informed of available options to relieve your suffering, including palliative care; and
- have waited 90 days before receiving MAID if your medical condition is "chronic" (and related to "Track 2"), rather than one in which your natural death is reasonably foreseeable ("Track 1").

At first glance, the medical criteria and safeguards for MAID may seem daunting. While they are intended to create a rigorous system of eligibility—MAID is not simply a rubber-stamp process—this can feel overwhelming, especially when you are dealing with a recent difficult diagnosis or a new stage of advanced, irreversible decline in a chronic disease. However, carefully considering the criteria and discussing them with a MAID provider can clarify the process and better prepare you to make important decisions.

## Eligibility Criteria: Serious and Incurable Medical Condition

To qualify for MAID, you must be suffering from a serious and incurable medical condition. Dozens of conditions may qualify. The most common types underlying MAID requests, and their prevalence in the 16,499 MAID provisions in 2024, are listed here [note: figures sum to more than 100 percent because patients could have multiple conditions]:

- Cancer: 10,065 (61 percent) (lung, colorectal, hematological, pancreatic, etc.)
- Cardiovascular: 2,799 (17 percent) (congestive heart failure, atrial fibrillation, vasculopathy, etc.)
- Neurodegenerative conditions: 2,278 (14 percent) (Parkinson's, Amyotrophic Lateral Sclerosis [ALS], dementia, multiple sclerosis, etc.)
- Respiratory: 2,222 (13 percent) (including chronic obstructive pulmonary disease, pulmonary fibrosis, etc.)
- Organ failure: 1,175 (7 percent) (kidney failure, liver failure, etc.)
- Other: 4,304 (26 percent) (frailty, chronic pain, diabetes, autoimmune conditions; also joint, bone, and muscle issues; hearing and visual issues; and various internal diseases, etc.)

As discussed in Chapter 5, mental illness, on its own, is not eligible for MAID until March 2027. After that date, it will be eligible like any other medical condition (unless the federal government extends the exception). Even before this date, mental illness can be considered for MAID if it is present alongside one or more other medical conditions.

To access MAID, your medical condition must be incurable, generally meaning one of two things: first, there is no cure for your condition, or none that is reasonably accessible to you in your province. The MAID provider performing your assessment determines a disorder's "curability." However, you ultimately decide whether a proposed treatment is reasonable given your circumstances; for example, it might involve discomfort, pain, or suffering that is unacceptable to you. For instance, refusing chemotherapy for a cancer with a 50 percent chance of full recovery might be unreasonable for a fifty-five-year-old. In contrast, refusing the same treatment with only a 10 percent chance of full recovery might be reasonable for an eighty-five-year-old.

To determine if a medical condition is curable, and explore potential treatments, a thorough discussion with a MAID provider is essential. Together, you can consider the nature and prognosis of your condition, your personal goals, best medical practices for treatment (or declining treatment), and other relevant factors. This can be a complex discussion. In 2024, 291 individuals seeking MAID were denied because they did not meet the requirement of having an incurable illness or medical condition.

Frailty can further illustrate the process of assessing incurability. Frailty is a recognized condition typically involving loss of muscle mass and strength, cognitive impairment, fatigue, exhaustion, and weakness, often leading to falls. Frailty exists in varying degrees: mild, moderate, and severe. Studies show that some individuals with mild frailty can progress to moderate frailty but return to mild frailty with sufficient exercise and improved diet. In such cases, the MAID requirement of irreversible decline might not be met.

Conversely, studies indicate that it is rare for a person who has declined from moderate frailty to severe frailty to return to moderate, let alone mild, frailty. In such cases, the criterion for irreversible decline would likely be present. Therefore, considering other factors, someone with only mild frailty, or who has recently progressed from mild to moderate frailty, might not be assessed as incurable. However, someone who has been severely frail for some time would likely be assessed as eligible for MAID. For example, in 2023, 92 people were found eligible for MAID based on frailty alone. However, each MAID case is carefully assessed on its own merits. This discussion of frailty highlights why it's crucial to consult with a MAID provider early in the process, rather than attempting to self-determine eligibility, if you are contemplating MAID or are simply "MAID-curious."

## Advanced State of Irreversible Decline

In addition to having a serious and incurable medical condition (as discussed earlier), accessing MAID requires that your medical condition has caused you to experience an advanced state of irreversible decline. This decline can involve both physical capability and cognitive capacity. In 2024, approximately 90 percent of Canadians who received MAID were unable to perform most "activities of daily living" independently. These activities include getting out of bed or a chair, walking, using the toilet, eating, dressing, bathing, and grooming. It also includes the inability to perform higher-level functions (often called "activities of independent living") such as shopping, preparing food, maintaining a household, doing laundry, managing medications, making phone calls, travelling, or handling finances.

Also in 2024, the advanced state of irreversible decline involved the following for MAID requesters: persistent significant fatigue/weakness (approximately 80 percent); persistent, significant, and escalating chronic pain (approximately 58 percent); significant dependence on aids for interaction and/or mobility (approximately 52 percent); reduced or minimal oral intake or difficulty swallowing (approximately 48 percent); cachexia, which is unintentional severe weight loss or marked change in weight and/or muscle loss (approximately 44 percent); significant shortness of breath (approximately 37 percent); and dependence on life-sustaining treatments such as oxygen therapy (approximately 22 percent).

Regarding cognitive capabilities, such as in certain dementia conditions, an "advanced state of irreversible decline" could include memory loss (regarding the past) and/or a degree of cognitive impairment that impacts the ability to perform tasks or plan specific actions in the near to medium future. Furthermore, an imminent loss of mental capacity from dementia would generally qualify as an advanced state of irreversible decline, as the very proximity of loss of capacity indicates significant progression of decline.

## Intolerable Suffering

In addition to having a serious and incurable medical condition that has caused a significant irreversible decline, accessing MAID requires that you are suffering intolerably from the medical condition and/or the decline it has caused. Therefore, if you seek MAID, the provider will ask you to explain how your medical condition or the advanced irreversible decline caused by your medical condition is causing you to suffer. The following are causes of intolerable suffering reported for MAID procedures performed in 2024, with the percentage of MAID requesters who mentioned each specific example of suffering (the figures sum to more than 100 percent because requesters could mention more than one type of suffering):

- loss of the ability to engage in meaningful activities: 96 percent
- loss of the ability to perform activities of daily living: 85 percent
- loss of independence: 76 percent
- loss of dignity: 65 percent
- inadequate pain control: 56 percent
- inadequate control of other symptoms: 55 percent.

The following conditions contribute to intolerable suffering:

- Burden on family, friends, and caregivers: 49 percent
- Emotional distress, anxiety, fear, existential suffering: 38 percent
- Loss of control of bodily functions: 32 percent
- Isolation or loneliness: 21 percent

Note: For Track 2 MAID requesters, isolation or loneliness: 44 percent

It is important to note that these conditions of intolerable suffering (and any others) are determined solely by you, the MAID requester. Therefore, the test for intolerable suffering is "subjective," not "objective." A situation you find intolerable might be tolerable to someone else. What matters is how *you* feel and what *you* conclude about your situation. In Canada, a MAID provider must respect your views on the type and degree of suffering you are experiencing.

## Administrative Requirements: MAID Is Only for Adults

To access MAID, you must be eighteen years of age or older; in Canada, only adults can receive MAID. There has been discussion of allowing mature minors to access MAID, for example, when a fifteen-year-old has terminal Leukaemia and the parents consent, but these discussions have not yet led to a change in the law (as of April 2026). See the additional discussion of "mature minors" in Chapter 5 (a mature minor is someone under the age of eighteen who a court has examined and found to have the decisional capability for medical matters).

## MAID Is Only for Canadian Residents

To access MAID in Canada, you must be eligible to receive healthcare services from your provincial medical insurance plan. For instance, in Ontario, you must be either a citizen or a permanent resident who spends at least six months a year in Ontario. Therefore, "MAID tourism" is not permitted in Canada; temporary visitors cannot come to Canada solely to receive MAID. This differs from Switzerland, where residents from other countries can register with a Swiss MAID clinic, like Dignitas, to go to Switzerland for MAID.

## Safeguards: Second Opinion

In Canada, two MAID providers must find you eligible to receive MAID. If the initial MAID provider finds you eligible, that provider asks a second MAID provider to assess you for eligibility. This process is described in more detail below.

## Voluntariness

In Canada, only voluntary MAID is permitted. To receive MAID, you must clearly request it of your own volition, free from duress or coercion. During the MAID eligibility assessment, the provider typically asks everyone except the requester to leave the room to ensure the request is voluntary and not influenced by others. If the provider determines the request is not voluntary, the individual will be deemed ineligible. In 2024, forty-five MAID requesters were denied eligibility due to a lack of voluntary consent.

## Capacity to Consent and Informed Consent

In Canada, MAID is only available to individuals with the mental capacity to provide informed consent. During separate assessments, MAID providers evaluate mental capacity by asking questions to determine understanding of MAID, its consequences, and alternative options for alleviating suffering. They assess the individual's cognitive ability to process and communicate about these issues. In 2024, 425 individuals requesting MAID were deemed incapable of making informed decisions regarding their health.

Consent to MAID must also be "informed." Providers will discuss alternative means of relieving suffering, including palliative care. Notably, approximately 75 percent of individuals who received MAID in Canada were already receiving palliative care. Providers carefully observe the requester to ensure comprehension of this information. Each year, a significant number of requesters fail to meet this consent safeguard; in 2024, this figure was 306 individuals.

Palliative care, as described in Chapter 1, is an important consideration. Some view palliative care and MAID as mutually exclusive, but they are often used in conjunction. Patients may begin with palliative care and choose MAID if it proves insufficient. In 2024, approximately 75 percent of MAID recipients also accessed palliative care.

Consent must be present at the initial request and reaffirmed immediately before MAID administration. The procedure proceeds only if the individual confirms their desire for MAID at this final opportunity.

There is an exception to the above. If your MAID assessors foresaw a risk that you would lose the capacity to consent before the scheduled MAID provision, the MAID provider could have you sign a "Waiver of Final Consent" form. In this case, MAID would proceed without the typical final verbal consent given just before the procedure. However, the MAID procedure must be administered by the date specified in the Waiver of Final Consent form, which is usually in the near future. You cannot request or consent to a MAID procedure in advance under any other circumstance, except in Quebec. There, under a law passed in November 2024, residents can complete Advance Requests for MAID. Chapter 5 discusses the important limitations of this Advance Request procedure in Quebec.

Your ability to consent to MAID may be compromised if you have some form of dementia, including Alzheimer's; however, most people in the early (mild) stage of dementia can still make informed decisions about MAID. If you are considering MAID because of a dementia diagnosis, make this decision before you lose capacity.

In other words, if you are diagnosed with dementia, including Alzheimer's, you must have sufficient capacity to give informed consent regarding MAID both when you are deemed eligible and when you receive MAID. Therefore, if you delay scheduling your MAID provision and lose capacity (due to progressing dementia/Alzheimer's) before it can be administered, you will no longer be eligible (except in Quebec, as noted earlier, or subject to the "Waiver of Final Consent," which has a limited scope). In conclusion, if you are contemplating MAID because of a dementia/Alzheimer's diagnosis, promptly discuss the nuances of your situation with a MAID provider.

Robert Munsch, the well-known Canadian children's book author, provides an example of MAID planning around dementia. According to press reports, Munsch was diagnosed with dementia in 2021 (some reports also indicate he has Parkinson's). These reports also state that he underwent a MAID assessment sometime after his diagnosis and was found eligible. He then indicated in a media report that he was waiting for the point when he risked losing his full capacity to write stories, at which time he would request MAID. Presumably, he is carefully monitoring his ongoing capacity and will opt for MAID when he has suffered serious, irreversible mental decline but still retains sufficient capacity to consent. (Note that if he were in Quebec, the process could differ under that province's Advance Request system, as noted in Chapter 5.)

## Track 2 MAID Cases

Two additional safeguards apply to "Track 2" cases under Canada's MAID law, where natural death from your medical condition is not "reasonably foreseeable." For example, this would apply to individuals with chronic conditions like Multiple Sclerosis (MS). Even if you have experienced an advanced state of irreversible decline due to MS, or due to circumstances caused by MS, and are suffering intolerably from the disease or the irreversible decline—particularly if you enter a care home to manage symptoms such as the inability to walk independently—you would likely live for several more years. Nevertheless, as a Track 2 case, you would be entitled to MAID if you are suffering intolerably from your MS, assuming you meet all other eligibility conditions, administrative requirements, and safeguards.

Under Canadian MAID, this MS scenario would be considered a Track 2 case. Track 1 MAID cases are those where a natural death is reasonably foreseeable, such as a terminal, end-stage cancer patient. (However, Track 1 cases include many situations where there is no terminal condition, and MS cases are often treated as Track 1 cases, depending on the specific circumstances.) Track 2 MAID cases have additional safeguards that do not apply to Track 1 cases. First, if neither MAID provider assessing you has expertise in the medical condition underlying your Track 2 MAID request (i.e., MS in the earlier example), at least one of the MAID providers must consult with a physician who has that expertise.

Another safeguard for Track 2 MAID cases is a mandatory ninety-day waiting period between the initial assessment and the MAID provision. During this three-month period, your MAID assessors are required to fully inform you about, and explore with you, available alternative means to relieve your suffering. They must also discuss and offer consultations regarding alternatives to MAID, such as moving into a care facility. You are not required to try these alternatives unless you wish to do so. However, if trying a specific alternative is necessary for the MAID provider to assess its potential to improve your condition, declining to try it may lead the provider to deem you ineligible for MAID. Given the dependence on the specific facts of your case, a meaningful consideration of whether MAID is right for you requires consulting with a MAID provider.

## Oversight of the MAID System

Each province has a formal oversight procedure to ensure that MAID providers adhere to relevant rules and practice standards. In Ontario, for instance, each MAID provider must promptly submit a detailed report to the Office of the Ontario Chief Coroner (OCC) after each MAID provision. The OCC staff reviews these reports and follows up on any questions or concerns. Compliance oversight could result in referrals to the relevant Ontario college of physicians or to the police. The OCC also organizes a MAID Death Review Committee, which reviews broader issues, such as best practices for Track 2 MAID procedures.

## MAID by Age

MAID patients represent a wide range of ages. In 2024, the median age for Track 1 MAID patients was 78.0, with almost 40 percent being under seventy-five. The age range is even more pronounced for Track 2 patients. In 2024, the median age for Track 2 patients was 75.9, with just over 46 percent being under 75. Notably, 21.6 percent of Track 2 MAID patients were under sixty-four.

These statistics indicate that approximately 25 percent of individuals who receive MAID in Canada are between sixty-five and seventy-four. Considering this, individuals in their early sixties may want to initiate a general discussion about MAID with their family, as further explored in Chapter 2. Similarly, if you are in your mid-thirties and your parents (likely in their early sixties) haven't broached the subject of MAID, you might consider starting a conversation to understand their perspectives. While discussions about death and dying can be challenging, especially before a serious medical condition arises (as noted in Chapter 2), these early conversations are valuable to have with loved ones.

## THE MAID PROCESS

### Finding a MAID Provider

After carefully considering your circumstances, if you decide you would like to pursue MAID (or at least explore the possibility with a provider), your next step is to find a MAID provider to consult with. There is no substitute for speaking directly with a local MAID provider, as they can address your specific questions and explain the practical aspects of MAID in your community, including scheduling. This book can only provide general guidance.

In Canada, if you are at home (rather than in a hospital), there are generally three ways to find a MAID provider. First, inquire with your family doctor about their involvement in MAID-related services. Even if they do not perform MAID provisions, they might conduct MAID assessments. Second, if your family doctor is not involved in MAID, request a referral to a doctor or nurse practitioner (collectively, a "MAID provider") who is. As a third option, you can contact the MAID referral phone number, or general "health line," operated by your provincial government or healthcare system. Each province offers such a service, and the contact information for each province and territory is listed at the end of this chapter. It's advisable to pursue both options—seeking a referral from your family doctor and calling the MAID referral line—especially if your request is urgent, as either method may take time to connect you with a MAID provider.

If you are already hospitalized, ask your attending physician if they perform MAID assessments and/or provisions. If not, your attending physician should be able to arrange a consultation with a MAID provider, often from the hospital's "MAID team." If your hospital does not offer MAID services (see the discussion of "conscientious exemption" in Chapter 5), your attending physician should refer you to a MAID provider from outside the hospital.

MAID providers are in high demand, and it can often take two to three weeks to schedule an initial MAID assessment. In 2024, 1,105 individuals requesting MAID were either unable to see a provider quickly enough or died before completing both required assessments (dying of natural causes rather than receiving MAID). Presumably, this indicates that a significant number of Canadians experienced greater suffering in their final days than might have occurred had they begun the MAID process sooner. These statistics suggest that if you are seriously considering MAID, it is advisable to consult a provider early.

Upon receiving affirmative assessments from both MAID providers, you can postpone the procedure for a period, knowing that you can request it on relatively short notice. However, bear in mind that a MAID provider may require approximately seven to ten days to arrange the procedure (and in many cases, it could take considerably longer). In 2024, 1,502 individuals who received affirmative assessments died of natural causes before the MAID procedure could be administered. Again, this likely meant they experienced greater suffering than they would have had they initiated the MAID process earlier.

## The Initial MAID Assessment

After making the significant decision to pursue MAID and finding a provider, the actual process begins with an eligibility assessment. This initial assessment typically lasts sixty to ninety minutes, but may take longer depending on the complexity of your case (sometimes requiring a second in-person meeting). The provider will review your medical condition, current symptoms, and ask questions regarding the criteria discussed earlier, particularly concerning irreversible decline and the degree and types of suffering you are experiencing. They will also inquire about the safeguards in place, ensuring that your request for MAID is voluntary and free from coercion or pressure.

Throughout the assessment, the provider will continuously evaluate your mental capacity to make informed decisions (refer back to the earlier discussion on capacity, as it is crucial). If there are any doubts about your capacity, the provider may ask specific questions to clarify your understanding and decision-making ability. In 2024, MAID providers determined that 425 individuals lacked sufficient capacity to proceed. Again, it is worth considering whether earlier initiation of the MAID process might have altered the outcome for these individuals.

Typically, within a few days of discussing your case with your healthcare provider and reviewing your medical records—and potentially consulting with a specialist—the MAID provider will inform you of their eligibility decision. In some cases, particularly when time is critical due to your condition, the MAID provider may make and communicate their decision at the end of the assessment. Regardless, MAID cannot proceed until a second MAID provider also confirms your eligibility.

In 2024, 1,092 MAID requesters were deemed ineligible because they either: (1) did not have a serious or incurable illness, disease, or disability (291 cases); (2) were not in an advanced state of irreversible decline in capability (399 cases); or (3) were not enduring intolerable suffering (402 cases). If a MAID provider determines that you are ineligible, they might describe your request as "premature," and may suggest a reassessment in a few months, should you wish to pursue it.

If you are found ineligible for MAID, appealing this decision to a judge is unlikely to be successful. An Ontario court case, decided a few years after MAID's legalization in Canada, clarified that MAID eligibility is determined by assessing physicians, not judges. However, you retain the right to seek a new, independent assessment from another MAID physician. While uncommon, this option remains available.

## The Second MAID Assessment

As mandated by MAID law, a second assessment, conducted by a different MAID provider, is required. This second provider must be "independent" of the first, meaning they cannot practise in the same clinic. Furthermore, the two providers do not compare assessments until both are complete.

The initial MAID provider will inform you of the second assessment's results. If either provider deems you ineligible, you may, as previously mentioned, contact another MAID provider for a new assessment.

## The MAID Provision

If two MAID providers deem you eligible, the initial provider, or occasionally the second assessor, will contact you to schedule the MAID provision. You can proceed immediately or wait, as you prefer.

Scheduling typically takes seven to ten days, but can sometimes take longer, from when you express your wish to proceed as soon as possible. Keep this time-frame in mind when initiating your request, considering that in 2024, 1,502 eligible requesters died while waiting for MAID administration. The MAID provision itself is quick, but coordinating the MAID provider's availability, often involving a nurse, and dispensing medications from a pharmacy can take time, even after approval. Factor these timing considerations into your planning, based on your medical condition and preferences.

## Where to Hold the MAID Provision

You will also need to decide where to have the procedure. Generally, MAID can be performed in various locations, including your home, a hospital, a hospice, or a care facility. However, as discussed in Chapter 5, some hospitals, clinics, and hospices do not allow MAID on their premises, which may affect your options.

If you wish to donate organs for scientific or medical research after MAID, a mainstream hospital will likely be your only option in Canada. Organ recovery for research is generally not possible if the death occurs at home or in a care facility. However, inquire about potential flexibility in your community regarding organ donation, as there may be more latitude for tissue donation.

## Personal Arrangements for Your MAID Provision

You have some flexibility in deciding what personal arrangements you want for your MAID provision, such as who will be present to support you. Chapter 2 discusses available options. This aspect of MAID offers more control over the dying process than a natural death.

## Administration Options for MAID Medicines

The time has come in your MAID journey for the MAID provider to administer the necessary medications. You can choose one of two methods to receive these medications, which will cause your death. The most common method in Canada involves you lying on a bed (or sitting in a recliner) and remaining entirely passive throughout the procedure. Your loved ones can be in the room with you. An intravenous tube (IV) is inserted into your arm to administer the medication. The MAID provider will then ask for your final consent to proceed. Assuming you consent, the provider injects the following medicines, in order, into your vein through the IV:

1. Midazolam: a sedative and anti-anxiety drug that induces a light sleep (similar to anaesthesia used in surgery)
2. Lidocaine: a local anaesthetic that numbs the vein, as the next two medicines can cause a stinging sensation without it
3. Propofol: a much stronger sedative that induces a deep, coma-like sleep; this medicine can sometimes cause death on its own
4. Rocuronium: a medicine that stops all muscle activity, including the lungs and heart, ensuring death.

The administration of these four drugs typically results in death within eight to ten minutes. This method, known as "doctor-administration," has virtually no complications.

The alternative method is "self-administration," where you take the drugs orally. In this case, the MAID provider mixes barbiturates (such as phenobarbital) with a large dose of morphine (in powder form), a large dose of a cardiac depressant (such as digoxin), and a large dose of a beta-blocker (such as propranolol) in water or juice (the "medical mixture"). The MAID provider will ask if you wish to proceed. If you answer yes, the provider will hand you the glass containing the medical mixture, and you will drink it. This oral combination of drugs works to induce a deep sleep, quickly leading to a coma, while also suppressing breathing and disrupting heart function, eventually causing the heart to stop.

During self-administration in Canada, the MAID provider remains in the room to supervise the self-administration of the medication. They are also present to respond quickly if the patient vomits or regurgitates the mixture. While this is rare, individual reactions to the medication can vary. Successful self-administration typically results in death within thirty to forty minutes, although it can sometimes take several hours.

Regardless of the administration method, the MAID provider orders the necessary medications from a pharmacy, retrieves them, and brings them to the agreed-upon location for the MAID procedure. In Canada, provincial healthcare insurance covers the cost of these medications.

Doctor-administration is overwhelmingly preferred in Canada. In 2023, only three of the 15,343 MAID provisions involved self-administration. In 2024, none of the 16,499 MAID provisions involved self-administration. Furthermore, Quebec does not offer self-administration; all MAID procedures in that province are performed by a doctor.

## Death Certificate

You may be curious about how MAID affects your death certificate. Similar to a natural death, where the attending doctor prepares the certificate, the MAID provider completes the death certificate. This document is used for various post-mortem administrative purposes, such as probating the will and enabling the executor to manage financial matters. The death certificate will not list MAID as the cause of death. Instead, it will state the underlying medical condition that caused the intolerable suffering that led to the MAID request. This aligns with World Health Organization guidelines, which do not classify MAID as a cause of death. Consequently, Statistics Canada's annual report on deaths in Canada does not list MAID as a cause of death either.

## No Impact of MAID on Insurance Policy

Some insurance policies include a clause that voids the policy if the policyholder dies by suicide within two years of the policy's start date. While this clause exists in some Canadian life insurance policies, it may not apply to all policies, such as many group insurance policies. Fortunately, Canadian insurance companies generally do not consider MAID to be "suicide" if all standard MAID procedures are followed. For instance, if a policyholder with terminal cancer receives MAID in accordance with all applicable requirements, the cause of death for life insurance purposes will be listed as "cancer." However, standard rules regarding accuracy on life insurance applications still apply. This includes disclosing all known medical conditions when applying for insurance. Failure to do so could lead to policy cancellation, though the cancellation would be due to inaccurate information on the application, not because the insured person received MAID.

## Provincial MAID Hotlines and Websites

Contacting a MAID provider directly is the best way to get answers to specific questions about MAID. Following are the local phone numbers for the MAID hotlines for the ten provinces and three territories, along with links to their respective MAID websites (as of April 1, 2026). Please note that the ease of navigation and the usefulness of the information provided on each provincial website may vary. While these websites can be helpful, they are not a substitute for speaking with a MAID provider.

**Alberta**: Alberta Health Services
Call: 811 Health Link
Email: maid.careteam@ahs.ca
Website: ahs.ca/MAID

**British Columbia:** Provincial Health Service Authority
Call: 811 HealthLink BC
Call: 1-844-851-6243, Provincial MAID Office
Email: maidcco@phsa.ca
More information: search "Medical Assistance in Dying" at phsa.ca

**Manitoba**: Shared Health Manitoba
Call: 204-926-1380; toll-free, 1-844-891-1825
More information: search "Medical Assistance in Dying" at sharedhealthmb.ca

**New Brunswick**: Horizon Health Network
Medical Assistance in Dying Program
Tele-Care: 811
Call: 1-833-883-6243

Email: MAID@horizonNB.ca
More information: search "Medical Assistance in Dying" at horizonnb.ca

**Newfoundland and Labrador**
Labrador-Grenfell Health: 709-897-2350; Email: maid@lghealth.ca
Central Health: 709-235-1412; Email: maid@centralhealth.nl.ca
Eastern Health: 709-777-2250; Email: maid@easternhealth.ca
Western Health: 709-637-5000 ext 5168; Email: maid@westernhealth.nl.ca

**Nova Scotia**: Nova Scotia Health
Call: 1-833-903-6243; or in Halifax region: 902-491-5892
Email: maid@nshealth.ca
More information: search "Medical Assistance in Dying" at nshealth.ca

**Northwest Territories**
Call: 1-833-492-0131; or 811
Email: maid_careteam@gov.nt.ca
More information: gov.nt.ca/maid

**Nunavut**: Nunavut Department of Health
info@gov.nu.ca; phone: 867-975-5700
More information: maid.info@gov.nu.ca

**Ontario**
Call 811, Health Ontario; speak to someone on the "MAID Team"
More information: search "Medical Assistance in Dying and End-of-Life Decisions" at Ontario.ca

**Prince Edward Island**

Call: 902-288-1260

Email: pmc@ihis.org

More information: search "Medical Assistance in Dying" at prince edwardisland.ca

**Quebec**

Call: 811

More information: Search "Medical Aid in Dying" at Quebec.ca

**Saskatchewan**: Medical Assistance in Dying (MAID) Program

Call: 1-833-473-6243 or call Healthline: 811

Email: provincialMAIDprogram@saskhealthauthority.ca

More information: search "Accessing MAID in Saskatchewan" at saskhealthauthority.ca

**Yukon**

Call HealthLine: 811

More information: search "Find information about medical assistance in dying" at Yukon.ca

## MAID Support Groups

MAID can be a daunting experience, especially after receiving difficult news from a doctor or experiencing a substantial worsening of a chronic condition. As you explore MAID, support from someone who has navigated the process with a loved one can be helpful and reassuring. Several Canadian groups are dedicated to supporting individuals contemplating MAID, as well as their loved ones, both before and after the procedure.

These groups are typically staffed by volunteers with personal experience supporting someone through MAID.

MAID Family Support Society (MFSS), maidfamilysupport.ca: MFSS provides compassionate, one-on-one support across Canada, connecting individuals assisting a loved one considering or planning for MAID, or those grieving a loss due to MAID, with people who have lived experience. Their website offers a reading room, MAID stories, resources, and a newsletter. Volunteers are available to provide support by phone, email, text, or video call, depending on your preference. MFSS is a registered Canadian not-for-profit corporation and charity. Services are free, and donations are accepted through their website.

Bridge C-14, bridgec14.org: Bridge C-14 is a national non-profit organization in Canada dedicated to supporting people across all stages of the MAID journey. They support individuals considering or pursuing MAID, those supporting them, and those grieving after a MAID death. Their work is grounded in the belief that no one should face this experience alone, and that each MAID journey is shaped by its own mix of love, uncertainty, grief, relief, and meaning. Through facilitated peer discussion groups, shared stories, and lived-experience resources, they create spaces for honest conversation, deep listening, and connection. All support is offered at no cost, with gratitude for donations that help this care continue.

Death Doulas, eoldac.*org*: The End of Life Doula Association of Canada maintains a directory of death doulas who offer services to help individuals navigate the MAID process. These services include assistance with medical appointments, notifying friends, and providing a sounding board on various issues. This can be especially helpful for individuals contemplating MAID who lack family or close friends for support. Chelsea Peddle, a death consultant, has written a children's book, "Pancakes with Nana," to help introduce children, such as grandchildren, to the topic of MAID. Death doulas typically charge a fee for their services.

MaiDHouse, *maidhouse.ca*: Located in Toronto and Victoria, BC, MAiDHouse provides a comfortable and safe space, with attendant supports, where MAID can be carried out peacefully and with dignity. This is particularly beneficial for individuals in precarious housing situations. MAiDHouse does not charge for its services but welcomes donations.

CHAPTER 4

# CANADIAN MAID'S LEGAL FOUNDATIONS

To better understand the current legal and moral foundations of MAID in Canada, it is helpful to appreciate its history and how it became an important healthcare procedure. This chapter will briefly delve into that history to demystify the current MAID system.

## Alleviating Medical Suffering before MAID

Before the introduction of MAID, the options for those suffering from serious and incurable medical conditions were limited and difficult. Some people took their own lives (see Gillian Bennett's letter in Chapter 1). For example, Charles and Margaret Le Moir, aged eighty-five and eighty respectively, had major medical issues and chose to die by suicide, jumping together from their fourteenth-floor apartment in Victoria, BC.

In the pre-MAID era, it was profoundly undignified that people suffering intolerably from incurable medical conditions had to end their own lives by suicide without assistance. John Smith, who had Parkinson's, was unable to slit his wrists because of his tremors. He then shot himself in the head; his fifteen-year-old granddaughter discovered him the next morning.

Swallowing large quantities of pills was another common method of suicide for those with incurable illnesses. Nembutal powder, a brand of pentobarbital, was often used, as were sleeping pills. However, patients often lacked information about appropriate dosages and administration, leading to complications and unsuccessful attempts. In the mid-1990s, Austin Bastable, who suffered from MS, attempted suicide by drug overdose but failed. He later ended his suffering using a Dr. Kevorkian machine. Even with such a machine, because of the legal prohibition on MAID, patients suffering intolerably from serious and incurable medical conditions had to end their lives alone, which is incredibly sad.

Several high-profile Canadians ended their lives to avoid further suffering from serious and incurable medical conditions. In November 1986, Quebec filmmaker Claude Jutra, diagnosed with early-onset Alzheimer's disease, jumped from the Jacques Cartier Bridge in Montreal at age fifty-six (his body was recovered in April 1987 from the St. Lawrence River near Quebec City). In Ontario, novelist and short story writer Margaret Laurence, diagnosed with terminal lung cancer that had metastasized, ended her life at age sixty with a drug overdose in 1987. On the West Coast, Al Purdy, suffering from advanced terminal cancer, died in 2000 at age eighty from an "assisted death," though John Hofsess's assistance was concealed because it was illegal at the time.

Other well-known individuals, despite debilitating medical conditions, were unable to end their lives. Dr. Donald Low, Ontario's chief medical scientist during the 2003 SARS outbreak, released a YouTube video in 2013, while suffering excruciating pain from a brain tumour. He pleaded for the right of people like himself to end their lives with compassion and dignity, rather than needlessly suffering until their natural death; he particularly abhorred the idea of being carried from the bedroom to the bathroom. Dr. Low's video received approximately 30,000 views within two days of its release. He died in September 2013, less than three years before Canada's MAID system was established.

## Physicians and MAID: An Evolution in Attitudes

In the decades preceding the Supreme Court's Carter decision (discussed below), public support for MAID from Canadian physicians was rare. The Canadian Medical Association opposed MAID until the Carter case, at which point it adopted a neutral stance, allowing its members to decide individually. Thirty years prior, many doctors opposed MAID. When Oregon instituted MAID in 1997, physicians initially approved only one in six requests, and only 31 percent of patients received the required medications from their first doctor; the remainder had to consult multiple physicians.

Many physicians interpret the Hippocratic Oath as requiring doctors "to do no harm," which they understand to include any action that shortens a patient's life. Interestingly, ancient Greek society held a more nuanced view of individuals seeking to end their lives due to debilitating medical conditions. The Greek Stoics, for example, argued that if a doctor could no longer help a patient, they could provide a drug to end their life. Indeed, choosing death when life became too painful was a widely accepted part of Greek (and later Roman) culture: "If life pleases you, live. If life no longer pleases you, you have the right to die"—note that this is a "right to die," not a "duty to die." In other words, the Greeks believed that mere existence was not the goal; rather, living *well* was paramount, and "the wise man lives as long as he decides he should, not as long as he can, in each case as determined by himself." Again, note the emphasis on voluntary MAID, not involuntary euthanasia.

Palliative care physicians were once opposed to MAID, but today the Canadian Hospice Palliative Care Association is neutral regarding patient requests for MAID. Currently, palliative care professionals and MAID providers cooperate to ensure that each patient receives the end-of-life care they desire. In fact, many palliative care doctors also perform MAID assessments and provisions, and many MAID provisions take place in palliative care settings such as hospices. In effect, there is a growing consensus that palliative care cannot fully alleviate some end-of-life symptoms, such as certain types of pain, nor can it address the sense of lost dignity and complete erosion of independence experienced by many in the final stages of dying. MAID is seen as a way to alleviate these conditions. In 2024, approximately 75 percent of MAID recipients in Canada were also accessing palliative care.

## Pre-MAID Pioneers Who Assisted Others to Alleviate Their Suffering

Starting in the 1970s, several individuals assisted others seeking to end their lives due to intolerable suffering from chronic or end-of-life medical conditions. In 1975, Derek Humphry's wife ended her life in the UK due to terminal cancer. Profoundly moved by his wife's decision, Humphry wrote a book about it: *Jean's Way: A Love Story*. Humphry then went on to write *Final Exit*, which sold 600,000 copies in the United States. The book's central theme was: "I demand that I have control over when and how I die." In 1980, Humphry also founded the Hemlock Society, which distributed information about self-death techniques and advocated for MAID. This organization continues today in the United States under the name Compassion and Choices.

In Canada, John Hofsess, a budding filmmaker, was deeply affected by filmmaker Claude Jutra's suicide following his Alzheimer's diagnosis (as noted earlier). Appalled by the extreme measures people with chronic or terminal illnesses were willing to take to end their lives, Hofsess founded the Right to Die Society of Canada in 1991. He was also among the first right-to-die advocates to disseminate information about MAID online through DeathNET, which he started in 1995. Hofsess and Evelyn Martens also offered a private death facilitation service using their "Exit Bag" device, which involved a patient placing a plastic bag over their head and breathing in helium or nitrogen gas from a canister through a plastic tube. Similarly, in the 1990s, American Dr. Jack Kevorkian provided several types of "death machines" to patients with medical conditions who wished to end their lives.

Individuals like Hofsess, Martens, and Kevorkian risked their freedom by assisting others in ending their lives. In both Canada and the United States, assisting someone in taking their own life was, and remains, a criminal offense, except where a government-sanctioned MAID system exists, which was not the case in North America in the 1990s, with the exception of Oregon after 1997.

In 2000, Evelyn Martens was charged with manslaughter and endured a two-year criminal trial. At the age of seventy-three, she had to navigate the courthouse stairs each day in heavy shackles on her hands and feet, simply for attending an end-of-life procedure and offering advice on using the Exit Bag. Although the jury acquitted her, the ordeal was intended to intimidate her and others like her, including Hofsess, and the government tactic proved effective. Martens and Hofsess ceased advising patients seeking to end their lives, leaving sufferers to navigate the process independently.

Kevorkian was tried three times for assisting in suicide, and each time the jury acquitted him. However, after openly discussing his actions on the *60 Minutes* news program, a jury found him guilty, and he was sentenced to ten years in prison, of which he served eight. Like Martens and Hofsess, he ceased providing "death services" after his release.

## Canada's Criminal Code

Since at least 1872, suicide has not been a criminal offense in Canada. As well, in 1972, the federal government repealed the section of the Criminal Code that made attempted suicide an offense. In short, a person in Canada suffering from a medical condition who wishes to end their life can do so without legal repercussions as long as they act entirely alone (though, as discussed, suicide can be a difficult and distressing act, denying the individual dignity, compassion, and a death surrounded by loved ones).

While suicide and attempted suicide are not illegal in Canada, assisting someone else in ending their life is a Criminal Code offense punishable by up to fourteen years in prison. A husband wanting to end his own life can do so without legal consequence as long as he obtains the barbiturates himself and takes them alone. However, if his wife buys the pills, blends them, and prepares the medicinal cocktail for him, she risks committing the offense of assisting his suicide. Consequently, individuals who choose to end their lives by suicide (and who understand the law) avoid involving loved ones in the process or the final act, even as observers, to avoid casting suspicion on them.

Sadly, this meant that someone seeking relief from excruciating suffering due to a devastating medical condition often died alone. This is why MAID advocates like Hofsess, Humphry, and Kevorkian were eager to see governments establish legal systems for dignified dying for people suffering from debilitating illnesses. Still, it's important to understand that, even today in Canada, our MAID system only applies to doctors and nurse practitioners administering MAID; a spouse or other non-medical professional cannot assist another person in ending their life—even if that person is suffering from a serious and incurable medical condition—without facing potential criminal charges.

## Underground MAID in the Medical System

Before the introduction of "official Canadian MAID" in 2016, a practice that could be termed "underground MAID" existed within the medical system. For instance, in the early 2000s, a patient suffering from a serious, incurable, and painful medical condition might request a merciful end to their life. While the patient's doctor would prescribe a medium dose of morphine (often Hydromorphone) for pain relief, they might, in response to the patient's pleas, increase the dosage to ensure the patient felt no pain. The doctor would be aware that this increased dosage would also cause the patient to stop breathing, effectively hastening their death. This was framed as a "secondary effect" of the increased morphine dosage and was deemed acceptable by the medical profession. Some speculate that this may have been how Börje Salming, the renowned Swedish defenseman for the Toronto Maple Leafs, died in November 2022, ending his battle with ALS (as Sweden lacked a MAID system at the time).

Similarly, consider a near-death patient who can no longer swallow and is reliant on a gastro tube for feeding. If that patient pleads with their physician to remove the tube and allow them to die, the doctor might comply, knowing that this action will lead to the patient's death. Some physicians differentiate this removal of medical apparatus from actively administering a fatal medicine, deeming the former acceptable while rejecting the latter. However, morally, the distinction between the two measures appears negligible, a conclusion increasingly shared by physicians. Nevertheless, this distinction resonated for some physicians before MAID, and even persists in some cases today; furthermore, prior to the introduction of MAID, the law clearly supported this distinction. Ultimately, the current MAID system is preferable to the "underground MAID" of the past, which was conducted without accountability, oversight, or the ability to monitor for abuse. The transparent system of today is far superior for both patients and medical practitioners compared to the obscure practices of the past.

## Liberalizing Social Trends

Between the 1960s and the 2000s, several social trends paved the way for the acceptance of MAID in Canada. Organized religion generally declined, with secular lifestyles becoming more prevalent. Consequently, the Catholic Church, which historically opposed MAID (and continues to do so, despite polls indicating support among its members), gradually lost its ability to dictate societal norms on major issues from the 1960s onward. This secularization was particularly influential in Quebec's "Quiet Revolution." Even today, the Catholic Church's opposition to MAID continues to influence the discourse surrounding its acceptance (see Chapter 5 for further discussion).

The late 1960s witnessed the rise of women's rights, gay rights, and other social movements that persist to this day. In Canada, the federal government decriminalized homosexuality and instituted no-fault divorce in the decade following 1968, famously summarized by Prime Minister Pierre Trudeau as, "the government has no place in the bedrooms of the nation." Around the same time, the Liberal government in Ottawa began to ease regulations on abortion, which was previously entirely prohibited.

Despite these changes, Dr. Henry Morgentaler was charged four times for performing abortions outside the government's regulatory system. Each time, he was acquitted by a jury through "jury nullification," a process where a jury refuses to apply a law deemed unjust. These failed prosecutions sent a clear message to the government: "Stop telling women what they can and cannot do with their bodies." However, instead of Parliament acting, the Supreme Court of Canada effectively decriminalized abortion in the 1988 Morgentaler case, striking down the existing regulatory system as overly burdensome. This decriminalization remains in effect because Parliament has not passed new abortion legislation. Crucially, in its decision in the Morgentaler case, the Supreme Court relied on the Charter of Rights and Freedoms, which Pierre Trudeau championed for incorporation into Canada's Constitution in 1982. This Charter would later play a central role in the legalization of MAID in Canada twenty-seven years later.

By the 1980s, the "baby boomer" generation significantly impacted society, particularly with their desire to control all aspects of their lives. This included choices about education, work, spouses, family planning (number and timing of children), prenatal screening for abnormalities, contraception, and assisted reproductive technologies like IVF and surrogacy when natural birth was not possible. During childbirth, they sought control over pain management through epidurals and C-sections. For many boomers, this desire for control extended to decisions about how and when they wished to end their lives. By the 1990s, witnessing their parents' deaths, many boomers found the dying process unacceptable due to pain, suffering, and loss of dignity, even within the healthcare system, and vowed for a different end-of-life journey for themselves.

Concurrently, decision-making in medicine was democratizing. Physicians could no longer unilaterally dictate patient care plans; patient consent became paramount. Today, performing a material medical procedure without a patient's prior consent is considered assault, barring exceptions in emergencies where the patient is unconscious and unable to consent.

Growing public concern also arose regarding the medicalization of end-of-life care and the prolongation of suffering for patients with chronic conditions. Increasingly, patients were being kept alive artificially by machines like ventilators and blood pumps and feeding devices. Many worried that these technologies prolonged death rather than sustained life, imposing unwanted end-of-life conditions against the patient's express wishes. Similarly, the dying process and death shifted from homes to institutional settings like hospitals, nursing homes, and long-term care facilities, which rapidly increased in Canada during the 1960s and 1970s.

In response to these trends, by the 1980s, courts began granting patients the right to withdraw or withhold medical treatment. In Canada, this right was affirmed in the 1992 *Nancy B.* case. In the United States, the 1990 Cruzan case saw the Supreme Court rule that a patient could refuse unwanted medical treatment and hasten death by refusing food and water. However, the Cruzan court maintained that physician-assisted death would remain illegal unless explicitly approved by the state; at the time, no US state had implemented a system of MAID.

## Canadian Politicians' Resistance to MAID

Although liberalizing social trends in the decades following 1968 emphasized personal autonomy and self-determination in decision-making, influencing some legal changes, Canadian legislatures, with the notable exception of Quebec, showed little interest in enacting MAID laws. Between 1991 and 2010, nine private members' bills attempting to legalize MAID were defeated in the federal House of Commons, often by wide margins. For instance, a 2010 bill failed by a vote of 228 to 59, demonstrating Parliament's strong opposition to MAID.

However, the federal government did enact the Charter of Rights and Freedoms as part of the patriation of the Canadian Constitution in 1982. Two sections of the Charter proved particularly relevant to MAID:

> Section 7: "Everyone has the right to life, liberty and security of the person. . . ."
>
> Section 15: "Every individual is equal before and under the law and has the right . . . to equal benefit of the law without discrimination based on . . . physical disability."

In the early 1990s, some MAID advocates, emphasizing individual autonomy, argued that these Charter sections could be used to create an exception to the Criminal Code's prohibition on assisted suicide, allowing compassionate death for individuals suffering greatly from serious and incurable medical conditions.

## The 1993 Rodriguez Decision: The Supreme Court's Initial Resistance to MAID

In 1993, Sue Rodriguez, a forty-two-year-old woman with Amyotrophic Lateral Sclerosis (ALS), faced a difficult dilemma. Given her prognosis of fourteen months, she wanted to spend as much time as possible with her young child but also wished to avoid the harrowing final stages of ALS, both for herself and her son. Ideally, she would have chosen to end her life with assistance at the appropriate time. However, the Criminal Code's prohibition against assisted suicide meant that anyone who helped her would face a prison sentence of up to fourteen years. Without this option, Rodriguez would have to end her life sooner, reducing the time she could spend with her son.

To address this cruel dilemma, Sue Rodriguez, represented by Chris Considine, launched a legal challenge in Victoria, BC, (her place of residence). She argued that the Criminal Code's prohibition against assisted death violated the Charter on two grounds. First, it infringed upon Section 7 by denying her the right to determine when she would die. Second, it contravened Section 15 because it discriminated against individuals with disabilities who, nearing the end of their natural lives, were unable to end their lives as an able-bodied person could. Both the trial judge and the BC Court of Appeal ruled against her.

Rodriguez then appealed to the Supreme Court of Canada. In a narrow five-four decision, the majority of the court concluded that the legal system must unconditionally uphold the principle of the sanctity of life. Therefore, the state could not risk allowing individuals to assist others in ending their lives under any circumstances. The court emphasized that this was especially applicable to those nearing the end of life, as they were particularly vulnerable to coercion. Indeed, protecting the vulnerable is a central theme in the majority's decision in the Rodriguez case. Furthermore, regarding the Section 7 Charter claim, the majority in Rodriguez maintained that the right to life does not encompass the right to determine one's death, again underscoring the importance of the sanctity of life within Canada's legal framework.

The majority of the court remained unconvinced that an exception to the blanket prohibition against assisted death was feasible, fearing that society would inevitably descend a slippery slope toward involuntary euthanasia. The majority noted that no other country had a system of medical assistance in dying, and all major medical associations in Canada (and the United States) at the time opposed its legalization. The majority conceded that their decision would cause suffering for some individuals (like Sue Rodriguez) but maintained that this was the price society had to pay to signal the government's disapproval of any form of assisted death.

The minority members of the Court in the Rodriguez case registered various dissents, advocating for an exception to the assisted death offense for individuals suffering from a serious and incurable medical condition, such as Sue Rodriguez. The minority, particularly Justice Beverley McLachlin, contended that safeguards could be implemented to protect vulnerable individuals from involuntary death within a system of medical assistance in dying, thereby affording a compassionate death to those suffering from a serious and incurable medical condition. Justice McLachlin concluded that only such a system would align with Section 7 of the Charter, given that "security of the person" grants autonomy and self-determination to each individual to make choices regarding their own bodies.

In his dissent, then Chief Justice Antonio Lamer found that the prohibition against assisted death in the Criminal Code violated Section 15 of the Charter. He argued that it deprived disabled individuals, as their physical capabilities diminished, of the ability to end their lives in the same way as non-disabled individuals. However, judicial dissents have no legal effect, although they are sometimes followed in later court decisions. This was ultimately the fate of the dissents in the Rodriguez case, but not for a couple of decades.

Ironically, Sue Rodriguez had a doctor help her end her life after the Supreme Court decision, and she died on February 12, 1994, in the presence of friends, including NDP Member of Parliament Svend

Robinson. The British Columbia government's law enforcement arm did not charge the doctor who assisted Rodriguez.

Two years after the Supreme Court's decision in Rodriguez, Parliamentary hearings on medical assistance in dying were held in Ottawa. However, the committee did not recommend that the government introduce a MAID system. Still, like the minority in the Rodriguez case, some committee members called for a MAID system with sufficient safeguards to be an exception to the Criminal Code prohibition on assisted death. The minority positions in the 1993 Rodriguez Supreme Court case and the 1995 Parliamentary Report were ignored for two decades until the Supreme Court of Canada, in its later Carter decision, adopted the minority proposal from the 1995 Parliamentary Report for a system of safeguards for MAID and made it the law. This exemplifies how law reform often works in Canada: as a dialogue between the legislative and judicial branches of the government, and, in this case, as a conversation over time between the minority opinions in one case and the majority decision in a subsequent case.

## The Carter Decision

In the three decades after the Charter became law in Canada, plaintiffs successfully overturned numerous long-standing legal prohibitions because they contravened Charter rights. By 2011, the constitutional lawyer Joseph Arvay believed it was worth another attempt to challenge the Criminal Code's complete ban on MAID for individuals suffering from serious and incurable medical conditions. Public opinion polls had long indicated solid majority support for MAID; an Angus Reid poll at the time of the Carter decision showed 67 percent in favour and 23 percent opposed.

Arvay, who had used a wheelchair since a car accident in his teens, worked with a team of MAID advocates to bring forward a case on behalf of Lee Carter, whose mother, Kay Carter, suffered from chronic spinal stenosis. Before MAID was legal in Canada, Kay had chosen to travel to a MAID clinic in Switzerland to end her suffering, and Lee accompanied her. Because Lee assisted her mother, she risked prosecution under Canadian law, which gave her standing as the lead plaintiff in the case challenging Canada's continuing ban on MAID.

Arvay argued that MAID systems in the Netherlands, Belgium, and Oregon (established since the Rodriguez decision) demonstrated that safeguards ensured compassionate dying with dignity models did not lead to a slippery slope, threatening vulnerable end-of-life or chronic condition patients with involuntary euthanasia. The trial judge in the Carter case, Madame Justice Lynn Smith, reviewed the evidence presented by Arvay and in 2012 delivered a 1,400-paragraph, 395-page judgment. She approved an exception to the Criminal Code's prohibition on assisted suicide, allowing healthcare professionals to administer assisted death, following a rigorous safety protocol and only in response to a voluntary request from someone with full mental capacity suffering from a grievous and irremediable medical condition.

Around this time, a Quebec politician, Véronique Hivon, championed a right-to-die legislative proposal in the Quebec National Assembly. Following a broadly based consultation with the Quebec public, which began in 2009, and the Ménard Report in January 2013, Quebec politicians considered and ultimately passed MAID legislation that took effect on December 10, 2015. However, it had an important limitation: it applied only to persons who were at the "end-of-life."

While Quebec contemplated its draft MAID law, the Carter trial decision was appealed to the BC Court of Appeal (where it was overturned in a two-to-one decision) and ultimately to the Supreme Court.

On February 6, 2015, in a unanimous decision, the Court in the Carter case held that Section 7 of the Charter required an exception to the Criminal Code's assisted suicide provision. This exception would allow a person suffering intolerably from a grievous and irremediable medical condition to access medical assistance in dying if they expressly requested it.

The core finding in Carter was that Section 7 of the Charter protected the right to life but did not mandate a duty to live. Two decades after the Supreme Court decision in Rodriguez, the minority opinions in that case, as well as the minority recommendations in the 1995 Parliamentary report, became law. In its Carter decision, the Supreme Court found that an exception should exist in criminal law for competent adults with grievous and irremediable medical conditions who voluntarily request medical assistance in dying (MAID) from a healthcare professional.

## Bill C-14: Canada's First Federal MAID Law

In Carter, the Supreme Court delayed the effective date of its decision by one year. This allowed the Canadian government to implement MAID legislation reflecting the decision's main requirements and addressing subsidiary matters. The twelve-month pause also enabled the provinces, responsible for healthcare delivery, to prepare for the new MAID system. Consequently, Ottawa introduced Bill C-14, which became the MAID law implementing the Supreme Court's Carter decision.

One provision in Bill C-14 proved controversial. Groups opposed to MAID lobbied the federal government, arguing that if assisted dying were permitted in Canada, it should apply only to individuals whose natural death was reasonably foreseeable. Some government members also supported this condition, leading to its inclusion as an eligibility criterion in Bill C-14. This limitation, however, was absent from the Supreme Court's decision in Carter. Nevertheless, Canada's Bill C-14 became law on June 17, 2016. After that date, MAID providers began administering MAID to eligible patients whose natural death was reasonably foreseeable, mirroring the "end-of-life" condition in Quebec's MAID law.

## The Truchon Decision

In Quebec, Jean Truchon and Nicole Gladu challenged the federal and Quebec governments, arguing that the "natural death reasonably foreseeable" requirement in the federal MAID law and the "end-of-life" requirement in Quebec's MAID law violated the Charter and contradicted the Supreme Court's decision in Carter. Truchon suffered from spastic cerebral palsy, and Gladu had post-polio syndrome. Both sought the option of MAID if their suffering became intolerable. They feared the "natural death reasonably foreseeable" restriction would block them, as their chronic conditions meant their natural deaths were not reasonably foreseeable (under the federal MAID law), nor did they meet the "end-of-life" circumstances (under the Quebec MAID law).

On September 11, 2019, the court in Truchon ruled in favour of the plaintiffs, deciding that the "natural death be reasonably foreseeable" restriction should be struck from Canada's MAID law. The court also determined that a similar restriction in the Quebec law, which limited MAID to cases where death was imminent, should be severed from that statute. Neither the federal government nor the Quebec government appealed the Truchon decision; instead, they both amended their respective MAID laws to reflect the court's ruling.

## Bill C-7: Canada's Current MAID Law

To align Canada's MAID law with the Truchon decision, Ottawa introduced Bill C-7. This bill superseded the previous MAID legislation and became Canada's current (as of April 2026) MAID statute on March 17, 2021. Consistent with the Truchon decision, Bill C-7 repealed the "natural death be reasonably foreseeable" restriction as an eligibility requirement for MAID. However, it stipulated that patients whose death was not reasonably foreseeable (now referred to as "Track 2" MAID requesters) must be subject to several additional safeguards when accessing MAID, as discussed in Chapter 3.

## Canadian MAID Relative to MAID in Other Countries

MAID systems have been enacted in approximately twenty jurisdictions worldwide, including twelve states in the United States. Among the early adopters of legal rules for MAID were Belgium, the Netherlands, and Switzerland, the latter having perhaps the most liberal regime. Switzerland even permits citizens from foreign countries to travel to a clinic there and end their lives through assisted death if they are suffering intolerably from a medical condition, though they must self-administer the medication and cannot have a physician inject it intravenously. As mentioned earlier, Kay Carter utilized this self-administration procedure at the Dignitas Clinic in Switzerland.

Prior to 2002, the Netherlands and Belgium had judge-made legal regimes governing MAID. In 2002, both countries enacted laws that implemented stringent reporting and oversight mechanisms for physicians administering MAID. Generally, the Dutch and Belgian systems for MAID are similar to Canada's model, but with a few important differences. Critically, all three models focus on enabling personal autonomy in end-of-life and chronic medical condition decisions where the patient is enduring significant suffering.

On the other hand, Canadian MAID differs significantly from the "Medical Aid in Dying" (MAiD) laws in twelve US states (California, Colorado, Delaware, Hawaii, Illinois, Maine, Montana, New Jersey, New Mexico, Oregon, Vermont, Washington, D.C., and Washington). For instance, Oregon's MAiD law, the first in the United States and a model for many other states, prioritizes a terminal prognosis (less than six months to live) rather than the alleviation of enduring suffering. In effect, US MAiD laws are limited to end-of-life circumstances and do not apply to chronic conditions like MS, Alzheimer's, or other neurodegenerative diseases that cause dementia.

Another key difference is that US MAiD laws only permit self-administration of medication, not doctor-administered drugs (e.g., through an IV). The patient consults a doctor, and if deemed competent and having a prognosis of fewer than six months, receives a prescription for the required drugs, typically Nembutal, a brand of barbiturates. The patient bears the cost of the drugs, around $3,000, and stores them until ready for use. At that time, usually alone but sometimes with a physician or someone from Compassion and Choices present, the drugs are mixed with water to create a drink that the patient ingests. Occasionally, the patient vomits or regurgitates the drugs. Death can take, on average, forty to sixty minutes, but sometimes longer.

Notably, MAiD accounts for only 0.7 percent of deaths in Oregon, while in Canada, the figure for MAID in 2024 was 5.1 percent. This substantial difference is arguably due to the features of the respective systems.

# CHAPTER 5

# CURRENT ISSUES IN CANADIAN MAID

While Canada's MAID system will be a decade old in June 2026, and many questions surrounding it have been addressed by courts and legislatures, some issues remain unresolved. This chapter will discuss these outstanding issues, as well as address criticisms of MAID, as a mature, high-performance democracy should always be open to hearing its critics.

## Mental Illness as the Sole Underlying Disorder for MAID

A significant current debate surrounding MAID in Canada concerns cases where mental illness is the individual's sole underlying medical disorder. As discussed in Chapter 3, eligibility for MAID requires that the medical condition be incurable. Some psychiatrists contend that mental illness is always curable, given sufficient time and appropriate therapy. However, what if an individual has attempted all, or most, commonly available therapies over many years, including rehabilitation, medication, art, music, group/family therapy, and various drug combinations and monotherapies, yet their mental illness, such as severe bipolar disorder, persists and causes intolerable suffering? In such cases, many MAID supporters argue that the individual should be entitled to access MAID.

Jane Hunter was one such person who was unable to access MAID despite suffering from an untreatable and debilitating mental illness. Her audio statement describing her condition can be found on the Dying With Dignity Canada website, referenced in Chapter 7. At seventy-five years old, she was anguished by her condition when she died "having taken matters into her own hands" (unable to access MAID), as stated in her obituary. This presumably meant she died by taking her own life, alone and without the compassion and dignity that the MAID system offers. It is hoped that the government will learn from this tragic outcome.

In the Netherlands and Belgium, countries with MAID systems similar to Canada's, individuals with mental illness causing enduring and intolerable suffering can access MAID. In 2024, 224 people with mental illness utilized MAID in the Netherlands, and fifty-five in Belgium. In these countries, the medical professions, particularly psychiatrists, have developed protocols to ensure that individuals with mental illness seeking MAID undergo rigorous review to confirm that their conditions are not amenable to currently available therapies. These MAID practices could potentially be emulated by Canadian psychiatrists.

In 2021, when the current version of Canada's MAID law (Bill C-7) came into effect, the government, at the request of the Canadian Psychiatric Association, postponed for two years its application to medical conditions involving mental illness. This delay was further extended to 2024, and now extends until March 17, 2027. Many proponents of MAID argue that this exemption for mental illness should not be extended further. Indeed, in August 2024, two plaintiffs, John Scully and Elyse Brosseau, initiated litigation against the federal government, arguing that this exclusion violates Sections 7 and 15 of the Charter.

## Advance Requests for MAID

A core principle of modern medicine is that, with few exceptions, medical professionals must obtain consent before administering treatment. This requirement is fundamental. Similarly, a patient can demand that a doctor withhold treatment or disconnect them from a medical device, even if doing so results in death. The seminal 1992 Nancy B case, in which a judge permitted a patient to be removed from a respirator (leading to her death), exemplifies this right.

Typically, patients interacting with the medical system are conscious and possess the mental capacity to provide or withhold consent in real-time, including cases where they initially agree to a treatment but later wish to discontinue it. However, circumstances such as a car accident rendering a patient unconscious may prevent this. How, then, can patients communicate their wishes to healthcare workers in such situations?

Two common methods exist. First, patients can create a written document, often called an Advance Directive, specifying treatments they do not consent to or treatments that, once initiated (perhaps while the patient was unconscious), must be discontinued upon discovery of the Advance Directive. Second, patients can appoint a power of attorney to make medical decisions on their behalf if they become incapacitated.

However, under current (April 2026) Canadian law, MAID cannot be carried out based on an Advance Directive or a Power of Attorney. The MAID law stipulates that express consent must be given both at the time MAID is requested and immediately before its provision (i.e., just before the MAID provider administers the relevant medications).

The current MAID law has one exception. After consenting to MAID by completing the request form, being deemed eligible by two MAID providers, and arranging a date for the procedure with the lead provider (e.g., fifteen days later), a patient may worry about losing capacity before the scheduled date due to their medical condition, treatment, or palliative care. In this specific case only, the patient can sign a "Waiver of Final Consent." This waiver authorizes the MAID provider to proceed on the scheduled date, even if the patient has lost capacity by then.

However, the Waiver of Final Consent cannot be used in the following scenarios. In Scenario 1, a person suddenly experiences a stroke that permanently impairs their cognitive capacity to consent to MAID. In Scenario 2, a person is diagnosed with dementia and experiences a steady decline until, for example, eighteen months later, they lose the mental capacity to consent to MAID. [Note: The eighteen-month timeframe is arbitrary. Individuals with dementia who are interested in MAID should promptly consult a MAID provider to discuss their specific circumstances.]

As of April 2026, a person in Scenario 1 would not be able to receive MAID because they are unable to consent, either initially or immediately before the procedure, due to the stroke-induced loss of capacity. In Scenario 2, a person could receive MAID until approximately eighteen months after their dementia diagnosis, provided they request it and undergo the procedure before losing capacity (assuming they have experienced a material and irreversible decline, likely the case near cognitive incapacitation). After that point, they would lack the capacity to consent. Because the exact timing of capacity loss is unpredictable, continuous monitoring (with a doctor's assistance) is crucial to ensure MAID is administered before capacity is lost. The timeframe will vary among dementia patients; each case is unique [see aforementioned note regarding consulting a MAID provider about individual circumstances].

Quebec's MAID law addresses Scenario 2 through legislation that deals with Advance Requests. Under this law, a Quebec resident can prepare a written Advance Request for MAID, but only *after* being diagnosed with a medical condition that threatens future mental capacity, such as dementia or Alzheimer's. This Advance Request can specify the circumstances that would trigger the right to receive MAID. For instance, one might specify: "When for two weeks I cannot recognize my spouse and children."

However, a significant obstacle exists within the Quebec law that could impede the medical system from fulfilling the wishes outlined in the Advance Request. The law stipulates that, in addition to the triggering event occurring (e.g., not recognizing family), the MAID provider must assess the individual immediately before administering MAID to determine if they are suffering intolerably. If the provider determines that the individual is not suffering intolerably at that time, MAID cannot be administered, and the person must continue living with dementia or Alzheimer's, even if they no longer recognize their family. While a spouse or adult child can request subsequent reassessments to determine if intolerable suffering exists at a later point, the individual might remain a "contented dementia patient" for some time. This situation would frustrate the original plan, as expressed in the Advance Request, to receive MAID promptly upon losing capacity or, for example, not recognizing family.

Given this possibility for dementia or Alzheimer's patients, the only way to avoid it in Quebec (and the rest of Canada) is to receive MAID while still possessing sufficient capacity to consent immediately beforehand. In the Netherlands, this approach is referred to as having MAID at "five minutes to midnight," where "midnight" represents the point of losing capacity. To mitigate the risk of missing this "midnight window," most dementia patients opt for MAID somewhat earlier, perhaps at "11:30 pm" rather than risking waiting until "11:55 pm," using the metaphor. Again, this assumes that a material and irreversible decline in capability has already occurred by the "11:30" time.

For individuals with dementia considering MAID due to intolerable suffering and irreversible decline, it's crucial to pursue MAID while they still possess clear capacity. Missing this window means potentially enduring years of diminished life with the very condition they sought to avoid. If you have dementia and are interested in MAID, promptly discuss your situation and options with a MAID provider (contact information is available at the end of Chapter 3).

A key limitation of Quebec's Advance Request law is its exclusion of Scenario 1, which involves sudden incapacitation, such as from a stroke or accident. The law requires a diagnosis of a serious and incurable condition before completing the Advance Request form, making it inaccessible to those who lose capacity abruptly. Consequently, individuals in such situations may face a prolonged period of suffering as a stroke victim, potentially including dementia.

The federal government is currently considering a federal Advance Request legal framework for MAID. Ideally, this framework would achieve two goals: first, allowing individuals to complete the Advance Request form at any time, regardless of their capacity status. This would ensure their wishes are honoured even in cases of accidents or strokes. Second, MAID should be granted solely based on the occurrence of pre-defined trigger circumstances (e.g., inability to recognize family). While individuals could include more detailed conditions in their Advance Request form, such as indicators of suffering based on demeanour, the legislation should also respect the wishes of those who, despite appearing content, do not wish to continue living with dementia once they can no longer recognize their family. This new legislation would empower Canadians with the right to an Advance Request for MAID, respecting individual autonomy and end-of-life choices.

In the meantime, one backup measure to consider is adding a provision to your Advance Directive for medical care (the document discussed briefly earlier, which differs significantly from an Advance Request for MAID). This provision would state that if you develop dementia or Alzheimer's to the point where you cannot recognize your family members, and you contract pneumonia (a common condition in dementia/Alzheimer's patients), the care home or any medical professionals should not administer antibiotics, food, or drink. Instead, you would be allowed to die through VSED (Voluntary Stopping of Eating and Drinking). This is not an ideal solution because a VSED death, coupled with untreated pneumonia, can be difficult for both the patient and their family members to witness and is not necessarily a dignified way to die. However, this must be weighed against the prospect of living for potentially a decade with progressive dementia.

## Mature Minors

Currently in Canada, MAID is restricted to individuals eighteen years of age or older, effectively limiting access to adults only. However, end-of-life medical conditions also afflict those under eighteen, such as paediatric cancers like childhood Leukaemia. These conditions can cause children as much suffering as end-of-life cancer causes adults.

Since 2002, Dutch law has permitted MAID for minors between twelve and eighteen under strict conditions and with parental involvement. Several Canadian Parliamentary committees have recommended a similar extension of MAID to "mature minors," provided there is parental consent. The current Canadian government is considering amending Canada's MAID law to allow some form of MAID for individuals under eighteen. A careful and measured proposal to allow mature minors to access MAID has merit and should be incorporated into Canada's MAID law. This would align with Canadian medical consent law, which grants mature minors autonomy in their medical decisions.

## Criticisms of Canadian MAID

In addition to the "open MAID issues" discussed earlier, various critics of MAID in Canada have raised several other questions that they believe require attention and corresponding changes in the law or practice of MAID. These criticisms are worth briefly discussing.

## Objections to Terminology

MAID critics often argue that the term "Medical Assistance in Dying" is inappropriate and should be replaced with a phrase that includes the words "euthanasia" and "assisted suicide." These suggestions are politically motivated. The term "euthanasia" carries negative connotations for many due to the Nazi regime's "involuntary euthanasia" program during World War II. Therefore, there is no reason to introduce a word into Canadian MAID discourse that would only serve to obfuscate matters and frighten people.

Similarly, the term "suicide" in Canada commonly refers to the act of taking one's life due to a range of personal reasons and social dynamics outside the context of MAID. Annually, approximately 4,000 Canadians die by suicide, typically as a sudden reaction to an overwhelming personal crisis. For example, the suicide of a nineteen-year-old in a fit of despair differs greatly from a seventy-seven-year-old choosing MAID due to terminal cancer and a limited life expectancy.

In other words, "suicide" is a social issue that governments actively try to prevent through various public programs. In contrast, in 2024, 16,499 people in Canada ended their lives through MAID because they were suffering intolerably from an incurable disease or medical condition. These two practices, suicide and MAID, stem from different motivations and dynamics, and the government responds to them differently. Conflating these practices, as critics of MAID often do, is unhelpful.

## Medical Professionals Raising MAID with Patients

Some critics of Canadian MAID object when a medical professional introduces the subject of MAID to a patient before the patient raises it themselves. This prompts the question whether medical professionals should be allowed to initiate the discussion of MAID with a patient.

This question has already been addressed. According to the federal government's "Standard of Practice" regarding MAID, medical professionals are not only entitled to raise MAID with a patient when appropriate (i.e., when the patient's condition suggests MAID as a potential option), but they also have a professional obligation to do so.

The reasoning behind this is relatively straightforward. For instance, when a physician informs a patient that their cancer has reached "end stage" and is incurable, they are required to discuss the various options available. The doctor will invariably discuss palliative care. Simultaneously, the federal Standard of Practice directs the oncologist to discuss MAID as well. In short, the physician should discuss *all* meaningful alternatives with the patient.

Unfortunately, the media sometimes misinterprets a medical professional's raising of MAID as the government-financed medical system pushing MAID onto an unsuspecting patient. However, this is not the case. The physician overseeing the patient's care is simply discussing all available alternatives with a patient whose underlying condition makes MAID a realistic option, assuming the patient chooses to pursue it. This physician-initiated discussion is not only appropriate, but also obligatory under the federal Standard of Practice, unless the physician is a conscientious objector, in which case they must arrange for another physician to convey the information. This practice of required disclosure of MAID in appropriate circumstances should continue.

This current practice in Canada also promotes fairer access to MAID, especially among people who might not otherwise be aware of their rights. For example, in New Zealand and South Australia, where a doctor cannot raise MAID with a patient (the patient must initiate the discussion), the participation rate in MAID is much lower than in Canada.

## Are Too Many People Having MAID?

Some MAID critics assert that too many people are accessing MAID in Canada, arguing that the approximately 16,000 annual cases exceed the original intent, which was to cover only a "small" number of Canadians in end-of-life circumstances. Some critics even argue that the year-over-year growth in MAID cases demonstrates that MAID is "out of control." This criticism peaked between 2019 and 2022, when the average annual growth in access to MAID was 31 percent.

MAID advocates counter that such rapid growth is typical with the introduction of a new product or service, and that the growth figures in recent years appear robust due to being measured from a small initial base. Indeed, the year-to-year growth slowed to 15.8 percent between 2022 and 2023, and to 6.9 percent between 2023 and 2024. It could even be argued that the MAID figures are quite low. With only about 5 percent of Canadian deaths each year being hastened through MAID, it is worth considering whether many Canadians are suffering more than they need to as they confront their dying process.

In the context of this debate, it is worth comparing the total number of deaths in 2023 from cancer, heart disease, and respiratory ailments with the number and percentage of Canadians facing such end-of-life diagnoses who elected to have MAID due to extensive suffering:

- Cancer: total deaths, 86,647; MAID cancer cases, 10,035 (11.5 percent)
- Heart disease: total deaths, 57,890; MAID heart disease cases, 2,703 (4.6 percent)
- Respiratory: total deaths, 12,994; MAID cases involving lung disease, 2,799 (21.5 percent)
- Alzheimer's: total deaths, 5,231; MAID cases, 81 (1.5 percent)

These statistics might lead to the conclusion that the dying process associated with respiratory ailments causes more suffering than other underlying medical conditions. Consequently, a higher proportion of individuals with lung disease may opt for MAID compared to those with other conditions. However, a closer examination of these figures suggests that it is difficult to argue that there are too many MAID cases, even for respiratory ailments, and certainly not for cancer, heart disease, or Alzheimer's. Rather, provided the MAID system is well-designed, incorporates appropriate safeguards, and includes comprehensive reporting and oversight, the annual number of MAID cases is simply a reflection of need. It is therefore inappropriate to argue that these numbers are inherently too high or too low.

## Religious Objections to Canadian MAID

Organized religion has traditionally opposed MAID. The Catholic Church, for example, argues that life is a gift from God and only God has the right to end it. Therefore, hastening death is considered a sin, regardless of the extent of a person's suffering from an incurable illness or chronic medical condition. The 1980 Vatican "Declaration on Euthanasia" stated that "life is a gift of God, and that suicide is, therefore, as wrong as murder." The document further asserts that "suffering has a special place in God's saving plan," and some proponents of the Catholic Church continue to suggest that suffering is ennobling, often citing Pope John Paul II's intense suffering in his final years as an example for Catholics to emulate.

Similarly, some semi-religious philosophers, such as Margaret Somerville, refer to the "mystery" of death and argue that MAID diminishes this mystery and the sense of community associated with a "natural death." The rationale behind this claim is not always clear, but it seems to require faith, or, more accurately, a feeling, to fully grasp. Furthermore, some extreme religious critics of MAID use inflammatory language, such as claiming that MAID is the fifth leading cause of death in Canada. This is inaccurate because, as discussed in Chapter 3, MAID is only available to patients already suffering intolerably from a serious and incurable underlying medical condition, such as end-of-life cancer or a chronic condition. While religious extremists are likely aware of this, they persist in using this incendiary language.

Given the fundamental opposition to MAID by some religious followers, finding common ground with atheists on this issue can be challenging, particularly when the former believe their faith prohibits hastening death, even in cases of great suffering. In these instances, agreeing to disagree may be the only option. However, a practical resolution exists: under a voluntary MAID system like Canada's, religious individuals are free to abstain from MAID. This straightforward solution offers reassurance, as a "natural death" remains the default unless MAID is consciously and actively requested.

Conversely, religious individuals should not obstruct those who wish to utilize the MAID system and meet the eligibility criteria. A principle of "live and let live" should prevail, encompassing the individual's right to choose how they wish to die. Religious doctrines should not dictate general law for those outside that faith. It is worth noting that some reformist elements within certain religions are adopting more nuanced views on MAID. For instance, within Reform and Conservative Judaism in Canada, some rabbis and leaders support MAID for congregants experiencing immense suffering from terminal illnesses where death is reasonably foreseeable. Similarly, the United Church of Canada does not oppose MAID when used by patients whose death is imminent. Times are changing.

## Healthcare Professionals as Conscientious Objectors to MAID

While religious organizations were unsuccessful in convincing the Supreme Court of Canada to block MAID under the Charter of Rights in the Carter decision, the court affirmed that its ruling did not compel healthcare professionals to participate in MAID assessments or provisions. This principle is enshrined in Canada's MAID law as the "conscientious exemption."

The conscientious exemption in the federal MAID law has elicited diverse responses from provincial governments (responsible for healthcare delivery). Quebec permits conscientious objection, but only for individual doctors. All medical facilities in Quebec receiving provincial funding must provide MAID services. Consequently, these facilities, especially those affiliated with religious organizations, must ensure they have sufficient staff willing to provide MAID, permit external MAID providers to attend to patients, or have a system for effectively transferring patients requesting MAID to facilities that can fulfil their request.

Similarly, the College of Physicians and Surgeons of Ontario, the regulatory body governing doctors in Ontario, mandates that any doctor who conscientiously objects to MAID must provide an effective referral to a non-objecting, available, and accessible physician. This typically involves finding a replacement doctor and ensuring the patient requesting MAID is properly transferred to that doctor's clinic or facility.

However, transferring a patient seeking MAID to another facility can be dangerous, especially for those in end-of-life situations, such as patients in the ICU connected to medical devices. In 2023, Samantha O'Neill, a patient in the final stage of cancer, was physically weak when she learned her hospital didn't provide MAID. The hospital arranged her transfer to another facility, medicating her into unconsciousness for the journey. Tragically, she never regained consciousness, highlighting the risks of such transfers for critically ill patients.

This ordeal prevented Ms. O'Neill's parents and family from saying goodbye, causing them immense grief, and presumably causing Ms. O'Neill great distress as well. Consequently, her parents have filed a lawsuit against the hospital that claimed conscientious exemption, Providence Health Care (which operates Catholic healthcare facilities in British Columbia), and the BC government (which exempts these facilities from allowing MAID). Aiming to change the law and practice, the parents argue that while individuals can conscientiously object to MAID-related activities, hospitals cannot. They contend that even in a "Catholic hospital," if a particular MAID provider opts out, another staff member must be ready to provide MAID. In essence, only people can exercise conscientious objection, not institutions.

It will be interesting to observe the legal system's response to this case. In the meantime, it is crucial that individuals considering MAID understand the position of the hospital they are being admitted to regarding conscientious exemptions. When possible, patients may want to direct ambulance attendants to a hospital that allows MAID to avoid a tragic situation like Ms. O'Neill's.

Similarly, when choosing a general practitioner, it's wise to understand their stance on MAID. This avoids developing a long-term patient-doctor relationship only to discover, when you're considering MAID, that your GP opposes it. This would deny you their support and advice during this significant decision.

## The Critique of MAID Based on Lack of Income/ Social Supports

A secular critique of Canadian MAID centres on the argument that, because avoiding suffering is paramount, it is problematic that some lower-income individuals, or those lacking adequate social support, may be utilizing MAID when what they truly need is increased income and social support. In other words, with more money or social services, their suffering might lessen to the point where they wouldn't choose MAID.

For example, a 2023 CTV story highlighted Sophia (a pseudonym), who suffered from Multiple Chemical Sensitivity (MCS). This condition made her extremely sensitive to substances like industrial cleaners and smoke, leading to symptoms such as headaches, migraines, fatigue, insomnia, coughing, nausea, heart palpitations, and high blood pressure. Sophia lived in a below-market-rent apartment building operated by The Salvation Army. Her MCS worsened during the COVID-19 pandemic due to increased use of industrial cleaners and indoor smoking in the building. While the landlord attempted accommodations, such as converting her living room into a bedroom and partially blocking air vents, these measures failed to alleviate her suffering. Ultimately, she chose MAID due to the intolerable nature of her MCS.

Ideally, with unlimited resources, Sophia could have been moved to a single-family home, providing a much cleaner environment. However, neither The Salvation Army nor the government could offer this option. The healthcare system assessed Sophia's situation as it was, and she was deemed eligible for MAID because she was experiencing intolerable suffering from her medical condition and desired to end her life through MAID, especially since alternative solutions implemented by her landlord proved insufficient to reduce her suffering, as determined by Sophia.

Critics of MAID contend that cases like Sophia's demonstrate the federal government's true intention in establishing MAID: to end the lives of low-income Canadians through the healthcare system. This, they argue, would save the government significant funds in social support programs (such as income supplements and social services) that should be provided to individuals like Sophia. However, this argument faces three key challenges.

First, the federal government did not introduce MAID. As discussed in Chapter 4, the Supreme Court established MAID through its Carter decision.

Second, eligibility for MAID is determined by a requester's serious and incurable medical condition, not their lack of social supports, as illustrated in Sophia's case. In other words, lacking social supports does not qualify someone for MAID. For instance, 95 percent of Track 2 recipients with a self-reported disability were receiving supportive services, and 75 percent of Track 1 recipients were receiving palliative care at the time of their MAID procedure. No one in Canada can receive MAID solely due to a lack of social supports, including housing, disability assistance, or mental health services.

Third, regarding the "low income/lack of social supports discrimination" critique, the federal government's 2024 annual report on MAID (based on provincial statistics), like the previous year's report, concluded that the vast majority of Canadians who choose MAID do not reside in lower-income communities. Furthermore, media reports suggesting that Track 2 MAID recipients are poorer or more marginalized than average are misleading. The same degree of marginalization is observed among Canadians who die without MAID or those living with chronic illnesses. In essence, the evidence does not support the argument that MAID disproportionately affects low-income individuals lacking social supports.

That being said, in an ideal world, we would eliminate all suffering for individuals with serious and incurable medical conditions. However, we must acknowledge that such a perfect world does not exist. In our current reality, Canadian MAID, with its safeguards, offers a viable option for individuals experiencing intolerable suffering due to a serious and incurable medical condition.

## Access to MAID by Indigenous People

Similar to the previous criticism, another argument suggests that Indigenous people (First Nations, Métis, and Inuit) are disproportionately accessing MAID. This critique posits that the federal government sees MAID as a more convenient and cost-effective solution for addressing the medical and social challenges faced by Indigenous people, rather than investing in additional healthcare resources.

As with the previous critique, the facts do not support this claim. In 2024, 164 Indigenous people received MAID, representing 1.0 percent of all MAID provisions. Given that Indigenous people constitute approximately 5.0 percent of the Canadian population, they are not overrepresented in the MAID system. It could even be argued that their communities are underserved by MAID providers.

## MAID and Canadians with Disabilities

A third critique of MAID, arising in the fall of 2024, involves a lawsuit brought against the Canadian government by organizations representing Canadians with disabilities. They argue that the Track 2 provisions in the MAID law unfairly discriminate against Canadians with disabilities. These groups claim that Sections 7 and 15 of the Charter of Rights and Freedoms prohibit the Track 2 provisions, arguing that Track 2 endangers Canadians with disabilities. The irony of this critique is that the Supreme Court used these very sections of the Charter in the 2015 Carter case to establish the MAID law in the first place.

At the time of this book's publication (August 2026), little progress has been made in this litigation. It is likely that the case will take years to proceed through the legal system, including potential appeals to the Supreme Court of Canada. A future edition of this book will provide an update on this case.

## A Slippery Slope to Involuntary MAID?

Some critics argue that Canadian MAID will inevitably lead to a "slippery slope" toward involuntary euthanasia, similar to the practices of the Nazi regime in 1930s Germany. Is there any evidence of this in Canada? No.

Over a decade of experience shows that MAID providers take their responsibilities seriously, authorizing MAID only when the requester is over eighteen, possesses sufficient mental capacity, voluntarily requests MAID, and meets the eligibility criteria outlined in the MAID law (as discussed in Chapter 3).

Canada has operated a MAID system for ten years. As of the end of 2024, 76,475 people have received MAID. However, thousands of others who requested MAID have been refused for various reasons, as explained in Chapter 6. There is no indication that Canada is sliding down a slippery slope into involuntary euthanasia. Individual voluntariness and personal consent remain fundamental principles of Canadian MAID, and there is no evidence to suggest that respect for these principles is diminishing, let alone has been violated.

Chapter 6 discusses the hundreds of annual cases in which MAID providers deemed requesters ineligible, typically because they could not provide the required consent or failed to meet another criterion. These statistics do not suggest a drift toward involuntary MAID. There is no reason to believe that our mature, responsible approach to MAID, particularly among MAID providers, will change. Nevertheless, vigilance and oversight—foundational safeguards already built into the current MAID system—must remain important elements of Canadian MAID to ensure that we never slide down a slippery slope into involuntary MAID.

## Proposed Changes to MAID in Alberta

On March 18, 2026, the United Conservative Party government of Alberta introduced Bill 18 (the *Safeguards for Last Resort Termination of Life Act*), which, when it becomes law, would narrow the scope of MAID in Alberta in the following ways:

- restrict Track 1 cases to situations where the patient has a prognosis of twelve months or less;
- eliminate altogether Track 2 cases in Alberta;
- prohibit MAID in cases where the sole underlying medical condition is mental illness;
- prohibit advance requests for MAID;
- prohibit MAID for mature minors;
- prohibit healthcare providers from discussing MAID with a patient unless the patient brings it up;
- require a family member to sign the Request form for MAID;
- prohibit a healthcare provider from referring a patient to a MAID provider outside the province of Alberta; and
- increase sanctions for healthcare providers that breach Alberta's rules pertaining to MAID.

It remains to be seen whether this draft law, once enacted, will be challenged in court, as it seems to violate several aspects of the federal MAID law as well as the Supreme Court's Carter decision. Nevertheless, Bill 18 certainly sends a signal that at least one provincial government is keen to narrow the scope of MAID in their jurisdiction.

## CHAPTER 6

# FAILED MAID REQUESTS

Much can also be learned from the thousands of cases where Canadians requested MAID but ultimately did not receive it. To understand these "failed MAID requests," this chapter reviews data from the federal government's annual report on MAID statistics for the calendar year 2024 (the most up-to-date statistics available as of this book's publication in June 2026).

The federal government's 2024 report includes statistics on MAID requests that did not result in MAID, figures that offer valuable insights. A key takeaway is that if you are considering MAID, begin your search for a MAID provider early, as the two MAID assessments and the scheduling of the MAID provision take time.

More broadly, the data in this chapter suggests that each year, thousands of Canadians who desire MAID are unsuccessful in achieving a compassionate, dignified death for various reasons. If you are serious about pursuing MAID, understand that the Canadian MAID process, from the initial request through the assessment process to the MAID provision itself, requires time, and many people who delay their request are ultimately unable to receive MAID.

In 2024, there were 22,535 MAID requests in Canada, but only 16,499 resulted in MAID provision. Consequently, 6,036 MAID requests "failed." These failures can be categorized as follows:

- 1,327 MAID requesters were found ineligible
- 692 withdrew their MAID requests
- 2,017 MAID requesters died before receiving MAID

## Ineligible MAID Requests

The 1,327 MAID requesters found ineligible in 2024 were deemed so for the following reasons:

- 425 incapable of making health decisions (i.e., lacked capacity)
- 399 did not have an advanced state of irreversible decline
- 402 did not experience intolerable suffering
- 291 did not have a serious and incurable medical condition
- 306 did not provide informed consent
- 45 did not make a voluntary request for MAID

The first and fifth categories indicate a lack of mental capacity, which underscores the safeguard in the Canadian MAID system that each MAID requester must possess sufficient cognitive capacity (i.e., understanding) to appreciate the consequences of MAID and consent to it. It appears that 731 people were unable to meet this requirement in 2024 alone, raising the question of whether starting their MAID journey earlier, when their mental capacity was presumably more robust, would have yielded a different outcome.

The second, third, and fourth categories suggest that MAID providers are diligently ensuring that the MAID medical criteria are met before deeming someone eligible for MAID. This is encouraging, as it demonstrates that the Canadian MAID model is careful and thoughtful, and MAID providers are not simply rubber-stamping requests.

Similarly, the last category demonstrates that MAID providers are exercising due care to identify situations where the MAID requester is being pressured into opting for MAID, such as by a family member. As previously noted, an essential moral foundation of Canadian MAID is that it is only permitted for those who voluntarily request the procedure.

## Withdrawals of MAID Requests

The 692 MAID requests withdrawn in 2024 can be attributed to the following reasons:

- 196 decided not to pursue MAID after learning more about it
- 315 accepted other means to relieve their suffering (including medicines, neurostimulation, electroconvulsive therapy, and counselling)
- 55 were convinced not to have MAID by a family member, religious leader, or professional
- 227 withdrew for other reasons
- 44 withdrew for unknown reasons

The first category highlights that many people research MAID before submitting a request; however, some individuals only conduct thorough research while already engaged in the MAID process. As with many other aspects of the healthcare system, MAID providers must meet their patients where they are.

The second category aligns with the MAID model, where MAID providers invariably discuss with the requester whether they have considered alternatives to MAID. The third reminds us that while MAID is not authorized for someone pressured to have it, individuals with influence over the MAID requester can certainly attempt to dissuade them from the procedure. The role of faith-based groups should not be underestimated in these efforts.

## Died before Receiving MAID

A significant number of people who expressed interest in MAID in 2024 died before receiving it. The 2024 report categorizes these individuals, providing the median number of days between the official MAID request and the date of their death for each subgroup:

- MAID requester was found eligible but never chose a date for the MAID provision: 1,661 (45 days)
- MAID requester was found eligible but died before the scheduled MAID provision: 1,502 (19 days between request and death)
- MAID requester died before the two assessments were completed: 752 (7 days)
- Person referred for MAID or requesting MAID was too late: 353 (4 days)
- MAID requester lost capacity between the time of their MAID request and their scheduled MAID date: 107 (14 days)
- Operational issue blocked the administration of the MAID provision, including the patient being unable to be moved to a facility that allowed MAID: 34 (19 days)
- No MAID provider was available or willing to handle the MAID request: 12 (23 days)
- Other: 253 (27 days)

While the 2024 report does not provide patient-specific details, the first category may not be particularly concerning. Presumably, these individuals underwent MAID assessment as a contingency plan but ultimately chose a natural death, even though their death occurred, on average, forty-five days later. While they did not receive MAID, the MAID system likely provided them with the comfort and certainty they sought. In effect, MAID served as an "insurance policy" that they ultimately did not use.

The drivers behind the other statistics are less clear. They may reflect shortcomings in the MAID system (the stresses on the healthcare system likely extend to the MAID system) combined with inadequate planning and a failure to act early enough on the part of those seeking MAID. For example, the second category likely includes cases where the limited number of MAID providers prevented timely MAID provision, despite the individuals being eligible. However, it is important to understand that scheduling a MAID provision typically takes around two weeks (and sometimes longer) after eligibility is determined. As previously noted, if you are considering MAID, you should act sooner rather than later.

The third category also emphasizes the time required to receive MAID. People often underestimate the time (and effort) involved in a thorough MAID assessment. As noted earlier, MAID providers take their roles and responsibilities seriously and do not rush the process. In 2024, 752 people learned this the hard way and likely suffered more as a result. Similarly, the fourth category represents individuals interested in MAID who likely simply waited too long in their dying process. Again, if you are considering MAID, begin your inquiry sooner rather than later, as you may otherwise run out of time.

The fifth category serves as a reminder that patients must have cognitive capacity at the time of the MAID provision. These requesters were found eligible for MAID but lost mental capacity before the procedure could be performed, which is required immediately before administering the medication. If there is any risk of such an outcome in your case, you should sign a Waiver of Final Consent, which can be used to bypass the final verbal consent requirement if the time between the eligibility finding and the scheduled MAID date is not too long.

Sadly, the sixth category suggests that the MAID system in Canada failed thirty-four people. As discussed in Chapter 5, conscientious exemptions for healthcare professionals should be permitted, but institutions such as hospitals should not be entitled to such exemptions. Therefore, it should be government policy nationwide that hospitals and hospices affiliated with a religion (e.g., Catholic) be required to employ a reasonable number of professionals willing to perform MAID or, at a minimum, allow external MAID providers to enter the facility and provide MAID in a suitable setting. If this were the case, fewer MAID requesters would have their wishes thwarted.

Finally, the seventh category highlights that, as with other aspects of Canada's healthcare system, there is a shortage of certain types of professionals, including doctors and nurse practitioners available to provide MAID. These statistics emphasize, once again, that if you are considering MAID, you might consider starting your MAID journey earlier rather than later.

# CHAPTER 7

# ADDITIONAL CANADIAN MAID RESOURCES

The previous chapters provided a general overview of Canadian MAID as of April 2026. However, as noted in the Introduction, this book cannot answer all specific questions, especially those related to individual medical situations or family circumstances. To address these specific concerns, connecting with professionals in the MAID field is essential. Chapter 3 includes information on how to contact MAID providers and support groups. This chapter offers additional resources that you may find helpful.

## MAID Ceremonies

If you wish to create ceremonies around your MAID experience, several commercial companies can assist with organizing events or commemorations for a fee.

- Be Ceremonial, *beceremonial.com*: offers services to individuals in various end-of-life situations, including a specific MAID module (dated August 19, 2025).

- Kinwood Celebration of Life, *kinwood.ca*: specializes in creating visual content from photos, videos, and other materials to celebrate the life of the person considering MAID and provide comfort to their family and friends.

## Grief Counselling

Support may be needed to cope with the grief caused by the loss of a loved one. While many grief resources apply to both natural and MAID-related deaths, some organizations offer specific considerations for MAID.

- *Mygrief.ca*: this website offers a series of modules that guide you through the phases of grief. Module 26, *"Grief and MAID,"* focuses specifically on MAID and features short clips of real-world experiences from individuals who chose MAID or their loved ones.
- *Kidsgrief.ca*: talking to children about MAID requires different messaging than conversations with adults. The module "Talking about dying and death" provides guidance for parents discussing MAID with their children. It emphasizes the importance of early and honest communication to help children cope with the difficult news.
- The Saskatchewan Health Authority offers a written resource called "Helping Children and Teens Understand MAID," available at saskhealthauthority.ca, which provides guidance on discussing MAID with children.

## MAID Advocacy Groups

**Dying With Dignity Canada**, *dyingwithdignity.ca*: DWDC is Canada's primary English-language advocacy group supporting MAID. Their motto is "It's Your Life. It's Your Choice." Their website provides information on current MAID issues that DWDC staff and volunteers are discussing with members of federal and provincial legislatures, including those covered in Chapter 5. The DWDC website also offers helpful resources on a wide range of MAID-related topics, beneficial for those considering MAID or assisting someone who is.

**Association québécoise pour le droit de mourir dans la dignité**, *aqdmd.org*: as a province at the forefront of MAID, Quebec's principal advocacy group, the AQDMD, is an important organization. Their bilingual website offers comprehensive information about the MAID process and outlines the group's current advocacy efforts, including expanding MAID access to individuals with mental health conditions as their sole underlying medical condition, and to mature minors in appropriate circumstances.

## Information Sources

The Internet/Artificial Intelligence: the internet offers easy access to numerous resources related to MAID and the medical conditions that often underlie the decision to pursue it. AI services can also help locate high-quality information on these topics. For example, you can research what life is like with dementia or Alzheimer's, both before and after entering an institutional care home, or the daily routine of someone with advanced MS in a care home. While the quality of online materials varies, the internet is a vast source of information, provided you invest the time and energy to find reliable sources. AI can assist in this search; indeed, it may be useful to begin with AI queries and then explore the sources it suggests. However, as with all sources of information, especially online, exercise sound judgment to avoid misinformation.

Federal government, *canada.ca*: although the Canadian government in Ottawa doesn't provide MAID services, Canada's MAID law is federal (a section of the Criminal Code). Therefore, the government provides extensive information about MAID (Quebec also has its own MAID law). A good starting point is to search "Medical Assistance in Dying: Overview" on *Canada.ca*. This website provides links to sub-sites and specific reading materials, including the full 2024 report compiling MAID data for that year (the latest report available as of Summer 2026, when this book went to press), which serves as the source for most of the statistics presented in this book.

While the federal MAID materials do not include specific information for reaching MAID providers in each province (this information can be found at the end of Chapter 3), this reflects the fact that in Canada, MAID service delivery is managed within each province and territory's health ministry, as they are responsible for managing and providing healthcare. Contact information for these provincial MAID resources can be found at the end of Chapter 3 of this book.

You may find these government websites helpful. However, if you wish to explore specific MAID issues in greater depth, the following websites, hosted by individuals deeply involved in the Canadian MAID system, offer valuable insights and discuss the latest developments:

- Canadian Virtual Hospice, *virtualhospice.ca*: this website provides high-quality information about advanced illness, palliative care, and related topics, including MAID. To access their MAID content, click the "Topics" button on the home page and select "Medical Assistance in Dying (MAID)" from the list. Here, you will find featured content, articles, and videos. For children, they offer a well-designed MAID Activity Book that allows them to explore MAID-related questions at their own pace.

- Disrupting Death: this monthly podcast, hosted by Kathy Kortes-Miller and Keri-Lyn Durant, discusses a wide range of MAID-related issues with guests involved in various aspects of the MAID system.
- End-of-Life Law & Policy in Canada, *eoldev.law.dal.ca*: this website, largely the work of Dalhousie University law professor Jocelyn Downie, offers extensive legal and related analysis regarding MAID, including links to reports and other materials.
- Dr. Stefanie Green, *stefaniegreen.com*: as one of Canada's pioneering physicians in the MAID field, Dr. Stefanie Green speaks to diverse audiences about MAID. Her website's "media" section provides links to many of her presentations and interviews, offering valuable insights into MAID from an insider's perspective.
- Value Judgments, *valuejudgments.substack.com*: Eric Mathison (*Ericmathison.ca*), a professor of bioethics in Toronto, publishes this periodic newsletter about MAID topics, emphasizing evidence-based reasoning in MAID debates.
- MAID in Canada: this Substack newsletter (*maidincanada.substack.com*), created by Paul Magennis and Kim Carlson, British Columbia nurses working in the MAID field, provides evidence-oriented writing and draws on their lived experiences with MAID.

## Medical Non-Profits

Several charitable organizations in Canada raise money and awareness for research into specific medical conditions. Some of these organizations offer valuable resources on their websites pertaining to MAID, particularly from the perspective of the diseases they focus on. Two particularly useful examples include:

Alzheimer Society of Canada, *Alzheimer.ca*: in addition to raising money for research, the ASC supports people with dementia, their caregivers, and healthcare providers. The ASC website features an extensive section on MAID, emphasizing that it is a complex and personal issue. The ASC supports amending federal MAID legislation to allow Advance Requests. Alongside its support for MAID, the ASC urges the government to increase support for palliative care, high-quality community and home care, and long-term care, ensuring that individuals with Alzheimer's have access to a full range of treatment options.

Canadian Cancer Society, *cancer.ca*: while the Canadian Cancer Society's direct materials on MAID are limited (search "Medical Assistance in Dying" on their main website), the section immediately below, titled "Physical symptoms of advanced cancer," provides an excellent description of the physical conditions and resulting difficulties that many patients seek to avoid by choosing MAID. This is especially relevant for those facing an end-of-life cancer diagnosis where a natural death is reasonably foreseeable; as noted in Chapter 1, approximately two-thirds of all MAID patients have end-stage cancer as the underlying cause of death.

## Canadian MAID Professional Support Organization

In Canada, physicians and nurse practitioners who perform MAID assessments and provisions often belong to the Canadian Association of MAID Assessors and Practitioners (CAMAP). This non-profit organization is dedicated to training medical professionals who wish to become MAID assessors and practitioners. CAMAP offers its members intensive continuing medical education courses covering a range of MAID-related subjects, as well as a major annual conference.

While membership in CAMAP is not mandatory for MAID assessors and practitioners, the substantial percentage of Canadian professionals who belong to CAMAP demonstrates its expertise, usefulness, and influence. The CAMAP curriculum is accredited by the College of Family Physicians of Canada, the Royal College of Physicians and Surgeons of Canada, and the Canadian Nurses Association.

Although most of the materials on the CAMAP website are available only to members, some resources are accessible to the public. One of CAMAP's most valuable services is the resilience training it provides to MAID professionals. Delivering MAID provisions can be emotionally and psychologically challenging for practitioners, and CAMAP recognizes this by incorporating strategies to address it into its ongoing member training.

## MAID in Culture

Books, movies, and plays have explored the subject of MAID and related topics. These works can be valuable, even if they raise more questions than they answer.

## Books, Nonfiction

*A Good Death,* by Sandra Martin, describes how individuals suffering intolerably from medical conditions, including MS, Parkinson's, Huntington's, and mental illness, ended their lives before MAID was legal in Canada.

*Somebody I Used to Know,* by Wendy Mitchell, a fifty-eight-year-old British woman, offers a fascinating and poignant account of living with the cognitive decline of Alzheimer's. This book is highly recommended for anyone diagnosed with dementia or with a loved one who has dementia.

*This Is Assisted Dying,* by Dr. Stefanie Green, a leading MAID professional in Canada, recounts her experiences with MAID patients during its initial year (2016–2017), providing timely observations that remain relevant.

*The Last Doctor,* by Dr. Jean Marmoreo and Johanna Schneller, an Order of Canada recipient, describes her early experiences as a MAID practitioner, with valuable lessons that still apply today.

*Talking about Death Won't Kill You,* by Kathy Kortes-Miller, is an accessible guide to discussing death and dying with family and loved ones, including a chapter specifically addressing MAID.

*The Many Faces of MAID,* by Carol Cram and Cynthia Clark, presents interviews with seventeen individuals who had a close family member or friend choose MAID.

## Film

*No Way to Die* (Canadian, 2024) is a CBC documentary profiling Jane Hunter, who suffered from mental illness. Unable to wait for Canada's MAID law to accommodate individuals with intractable mental illness,

Jane took her own life in March 2024. An audio recording of Jane Hunter can be found on the Dying With Dignity Canada website (*Dyingwithdignity.ca*).

*Million Dollar Baby* (American, 2004) sympathetically portrays the mercy killing of Maggie, a boxer who becomes a quadriplegic after an accident in the ring. The film won four Oscars in 2004, including Best Picture and Best Director.

*The Sea Inside* (Spanish, 2004) tells the true story of Ramón, a quadriplegic after a diving accident that left him paralyzed from the neck down, advocating for MAID for twenty-eight years. He ultimately receives a merciful end-of-life from a friend. The film won the 2004 Academy Award for Best Foreign Language Film.

*The Barbarian Invasions* (Canadian, 2003) depicts Rémy, in his early sixties and dying of terminal cancer, receiving a compassionate overdose of morphine from someone outside the healthcare system. The film won the 2003 Academy Award for Best Foreign Language Film.

*Still Alice* (American, 2014) features Alice, a linguistics professor with familial Alzheimer's disease, attempting to take her life via an overdose of sleeping pills. The movie makes a strong case for MAID for dementia/Alzheimer's.

## Plays

*In 7 Days* (Canadian, 2024) by Ontario playwright Jordi Mand follows the patriarch of a Jewish family choosing MAID, which leads to deep and heartfelt discussions with a Rabbi and family members.

*A Question of Mercy* (American, 1997) explores whether a man with a terminal AIDS condition should be entitled to a doctor-assisted death.

# ACKNOWLEDGEMENTS

While writing a book is a solitary exercise, it always benefits from interaction with engaged and insightful people. I was fortunate to have Ken Whyte, a highly perceptive publisher at Sutherland House Books. I am also grateful to Mary Anne Cecutti, Jocelyn Downie, Jean Marmoreo, Eric Mathison, and Wayne Sumner, who read a "beta version" of the manuscript and provided detailed and perceptive comments. Any remaining shortcomings are mine alone.